the
GREEN
Beauty Rules

The Essential Guide to Toxic-Free Beauty,
Green Glamour, and Glowing Skin

WHAT TO TOSS | WHAT TO TRY | AND WHAT TO BUY

PAIGE PADGETT

Health Communications, Inc.
Deerfield Beach, Florida

www.hcibooks.com

**Library of Congress Cataloging-in-Publication Data
is available through the Library of Congress**

© 2015 Paige Padgett

ISBN-13: 978-07573-1870-2 (Paperback)
ISBN-10: 07573-1870-3 (Paperback)
ISBN-13: 978-07573-1871-9 (ePub)
ISBN-10: 07573-1870-2 (ePub)

Publisher: Health Communications, Inc.
         3201 S.W. 15th Street
         Deerfield Beach, FL 33442–8190

Cover photo © Don Flood
Beauty looks photos by Michele LoBosco
Illustrations by Yeva Babayan
Cover design by Larissa Hise Henoch
Interior design and formatting by Lawna Patterson Oldfield and Larissa Hise Henoch

This book is dedicated to my mom,
Diane, my first beauty inspiration, and
to my daughter, Marianna, who inspires
me to be better every day.

Contents

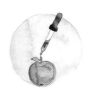

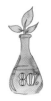

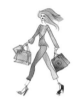
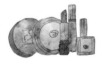
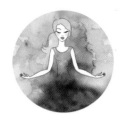

Foreword
by Jillian Michaels

Finally, a green beauty book written for the glamorous girl. If you're a person with discerning taste for glamour and beauty, but also care about your health and wellness, this is the book for you. Paige Padgett shows you exactly how to rid your beauty routine of toxic chemicals without having to make your own cosmetics or settle for substandard beauty products that don't work. No one is more qualified to show you how to be glamorous *and* green.

Paige has been my makeup artist for ten years. I have watched her go from being one of the first professional makeup artists to green her makeup kit to being a leading authority on chemically safe cosmetics. Her no-nonsense approach is straight-forward yet flexible, enabling you to rid toxic chemicals from your beauty routine and still keep some of your favorite products.

Prior to working with Paige, I had never thought about chemicals in my cosmetics. But Paige explained to me that just like toxic chemicals in food, toxic chemicals in cosmetics are just as harmful to your body. Since I was already eating organic foods and using chemically safe cleaning supplies and household products, greening my beauty routine was a natural final step in ridding toxic chemicals from my lifestyle.

> Paige has been my makeup artist for ten years. No one is more qualified to show you how to be glamorous *and* green.

Paige knows that women want to be healthy, look beautiful, and feel sexy. She knows that most women don't have time to do all the sleuthing she has done. In this book you benefit from her scrutiny of ingredients and claims. She has sought out quality products that are affordable. She takes all the guesswork out of it by revealing her favorite products and gives you enough knowledge and practical application so you can seek out your own. Paige will show you step-by-step how to green your beauty routine. She will empower you to make good choices for you and your family while keeping you gorgeous.

With something useful for everyone, *The Green Beauty Rules* is the green beauty book you've been waiting for, and I am thrilled to share it with you. Paige has been making me glamorously green and healthy for a decade, and now she can make you glamorously green and healthy, too.

Introduction:
The Green Glamour
Promise

Is it possible to be glamorous while also having compassionate consideration for our planet? Absolutely! For many women, greening our beauty routine simultaneously excites us and scares us. We want to do it because we know it's the right thing to do for our health, yet we fear it because it may mean giving up products we love or have grown accustomed to over the years. Plus, with all the misinformation out there, it makes the transition that much more overwhelming.

Fear no more! I am going to show you how to embrace a kinder, gentler cosmetics philosophy, one that rejects toxic chemicals and animal cruelty, without sacrificing an ounce of style.

As a professional makeup artist for more than ten years, I have eliminated chemicals from my cosmetics and have helped others do the same. I have also redefined my ideas about beauty and let go of old notions about so-called premium products and makeup as a symbol of status. It wasn't always easy to work with a green kit, retain clients, and attract new clients based on being a chemically safe makeup artist. Who wouldn't want to use what is considered the gold standard of beauty products, offering the widest range and the most beautiful packaging? Not me and not my Hollywood clients either. But, with persistence and passion, I've done it, and you can, too.

This book will challenge you to redefine your own ideas about green beauty. And the mere fact that you're reading this right now shows you're open to a new way of thinking. Thank you for being on this journey with me, and I promise to lead you every step of the way to greening your beauty routine. You'll learn how to make smart and sustainable choices as you move away from conventional beauty products to chemically safe cosmetics. Doing so will make you happy and keep you looking hot!

The first step in the process of greening your beauty is to understand what it means and why it matters. I didn't understand what it meant when I began my journey into living an eco-friendly lifestyle. I didn't realize that my cosmetics could have anything to do with harming our planet or myself. It was when I finally realized the impact of what I call my "cosmetic footprint"—my cosmetic toxic burden on my health and the environment—that I made the change for good.

As you read this book, you will come to understand why it's so important to use clean products on your skin and why I consider your beauty routine a diet. Skin absorbs cosmetic products like food; chemicals are absorbed through your pores into your body. This is why chemicals are so effective in prescription and over-the-counter medicines. You will learn what toxic chemicals can do to your body, where to look for them, and how to avoid the major offenders. I will teach you about the dangers of synthetic fragrances, parabens, and petrochemicals. When you learn how toxic chemicals react in your body, you will want to buy clean, nontoxic cosmetics. Buying premium brands won't matter as much to you as making healthier choices.

Once you start viewing your beauty routine as a diet, you will want to be cleaner in all aspects of your life. As a mom to a two-year-old little girl, it is important that I stay healthy and impart a healthy lifestyle to her. Since greening my beauty routine, I have made other positive changes. I feel more in control of my health and more confident in my choices for my daughter and myself. Maintaining glamour is the standard in my line of work, and I have been able to achieve and sustain a green beauty lifestyle that I am passionate about, where I look as good as I feel.

If you are learning about toxic chemicals in makeup for the first time, you're probably feeling overwhelmed and frustrated. I've been there too and I get it. So how do you know what's good and what's green? This is where the book comes in. I have spent years researching chemicals in cosmetics and using clean products with the goal of knowing what works and what doesn't. I know what changes women can realistically make in their busy lives, and I'm going to share everything in my vault with you. We're going to cover it all: what to know about the beauty industry, how to read labels, which chemicals to watch out for, and how to shop for pure, healthy, and high-performance cosmetics. I want you to be inspired by this information in order to become savvier, healthier, and sexier than ever!

You can read this book cover to cover or per topic of interest. It's laid out for you to achieve ultimate success. This guide will help you easily navigate the transition to clean cosmetics. Don't panic—I won't be asking you to dump all your favorite products at once. It's a gradual process. In fact, using my 80/20 rule, you may actually be able to keep your signature scent or go-to lipstick. Does that make you breathe a little easier? Hopefully so.

You can move between chapters as you need specific information, and you can go back to the book again and again anytime you want to find the best mascara or concealer. There are no hard and fast rules. Make it work for you.

So let's get started.

Chapter One

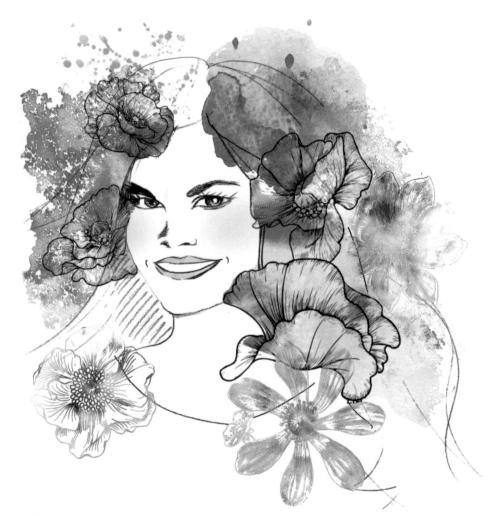

GREEN Beauty

Pioneer

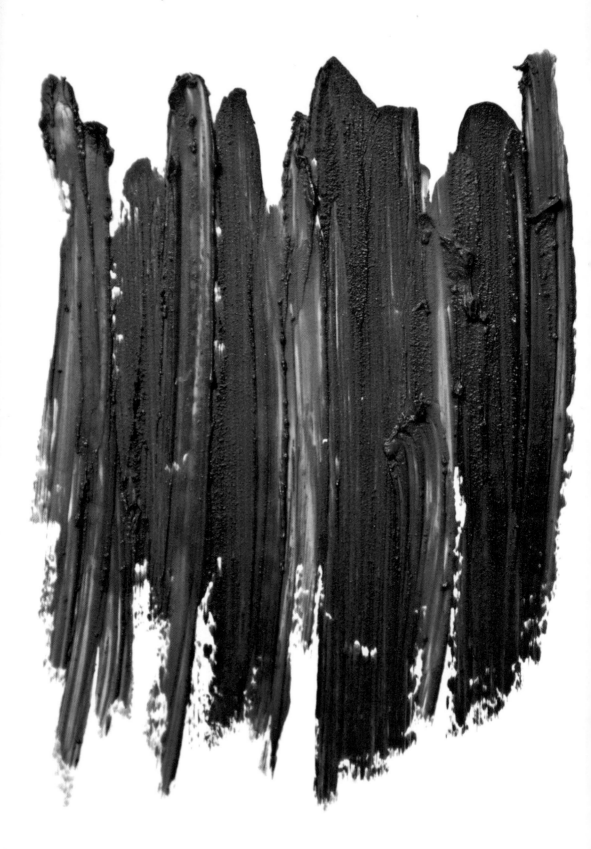

If I said I wanted to be a makeup artist when I was a child, I would be lying. I wanted to be like Phil Donahue or Sally Jessie Rafael (yep, I'm forty-seven!). I wanted to host a talk show so I could discuss pressing issues and help others. As I got older I looked up to strong women like Barbara Walters, Diane Sawyer, Christiane Amanpour, and, of course, Oprah, and dreamed to one day live a life of purpose.

Being a makeup artist never crossed my mind until much later, but looking back, it was my destiny all along. Over the course of my career I discovered that when you have passion for something and you work hard at it and never give up, you can be wildly successful and create any life you want for yourself. That's what I have done with my passion for makeup and sustainable living. I love what I do every day.

MY FIRST BEAUTY INSPIRATION

My mother was my first childhood beauty inspiration. Growing up in Modesto, a small town in central California, I was one of five kids. My mother was a single mom, and although we didn't have a lot of money, we always had an abundance of love. She was incredibly beautiful and loved to wear her makeup with a smoky eye. She still does today at age sixty-eight! As a child I watched her apply makeup in front of a mirror at the dining table. She liked to sit down and put on her makeup. For her it was relaxing and almost ritualistic. She always played music, too—usually Motown or disco. The smoky eye was her signature, and she skillfully designed it. It was the perfect mixture of gray and brown eye shadow. Unlike me, she wasn't afraid to be too heavy-handed either. Her pale blue eyes popped against the dark rim she created around her lash line. She was absolutely exquisite.

Just like my mom, I have adopted a ritual for getting ready when I have a special occasion. It starts with a long bath, if I can spare the time (not so much these days with a toddler!), and music, usually dance music or R&B, like Pink, Rihanna, or Beyoncé. I take my time getting dressed and putting on my makeup. It helps me feel sexy. It inspires confidence.

To me, confidence is what makes women beautiful. Have you ever noticed that some women can be in sweats, no makeup, and hair tied in a knot and still look gorgeous? There's a trend in Hollywood with female celebrities posting no-makeup selfies. The public response is that the women look more beautiful than ever. I love it because it shows that owning yourself and becoming comfortable in your skin is the epitome of real beauty. It's better than anything you'll find on the red carpet.

This concept of confidence and beauty is why I love working with Jillian Michaels. Yes, she is gorgeous, but it's her strength, determination, and self-confidence that make her such a strong force in the world of health and wellness. Not to mention crazy sexy.

MEETING JILLIAN MICHAELS

I met Jillian by chance. As I pulled up to the set of TV's *The Biggest Loser*, in Lancaster, California, a small, dusty town about two hours from Los Angeles, I only knew I was there to audition to do the makeup for one of the female talents. I was dressed all in black (my uniform), wearing sky-high stiletto booties and a leather jacket. I looked like I was going to a club, not to work in the middle of the desert. It was the typical artist attire for an editorial shoot but not a reality show in the hot sun. What was I thinking? In my defense, I had never worked on a reality show before. They are dramatically different than scripted shows and the culture and social norms are too.

Enter Jillian Michaels, wearing jeans, a T-shirt, and a baseball cap, very unassuming. Let me just say, it was the longest day ever. Here we were, doing her segments in the middle of the desert, and every time I had to smooth a flyaway hair or gloss her lips, I had to run—no, sprint—back and forth in shoes that could be used to aerate a field. I was humiliated as I made my way through the dirt, dodging cacti, gopher holes, and boulders. I felt like a supreme idiot and thought I'd never get the job.

Surprisingly, two days later, I was called back to work with Jillian, and we have never looked back. She is my client and my friend. When we retell the story of how we met, Jillian says she "laughed her ass off that day." I know she's not kidding. I heard her.

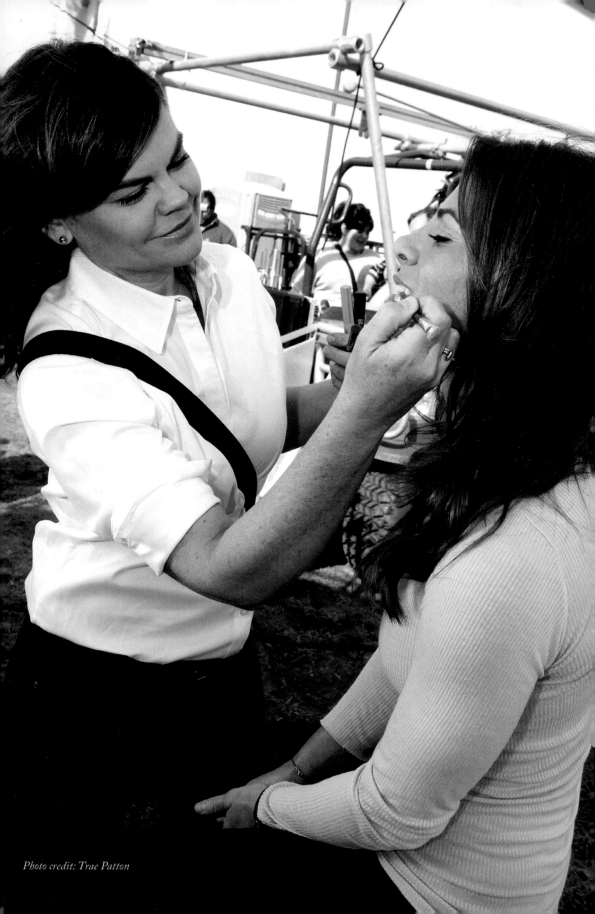

GREENING HOLLYWOOD (OR NOT)

While I was working on *The Biggest Loser*, I wanted to focus on honing my green beauty knowledge. I was still in my infancy with greening my makeup kits and knew very little about chemicals at the time. I was hungry for any information I could find to help me. I wanted products, information, and role models. When I searched online for "green," "natural," or "organic" beauty, there was only one other person doing what I was doing: Christy Coleman, an amazing makeup artist. There was virtually no one else.

Fortuitously, I had the perfect client in Jillian because she was interested in chemically safe makeup since she already had such a clean nutritional diet. She was supportive and graciously allowed me to experiment on her. Once, after training her contestants on camera, she came into the makeup room yelling my name, "Paaaaige!" Yikes! I knew it was the eye shadow. She hated it. She said that it creased, it was too shiny, and looked "disco." Ha! That's what I liked about it; I thought that wet look was sexy. But she was a trainer and wanted to look like it. It was a new organic line of cream eye shadows, and the colors were brilliant. She was right though; it would be great for editorial shoots, but it wasn't very practical for television.

Another time, after covering her from chest to hairline in a new natural foundation, she looked in the mirror and said, "I look like an Oompa Loompa." She was right again. It had an orangey tinge to it that was unmistakably reminiscent of those funny little guys. She was a good sport letting me test new makeup on her. She humored and indulged me often, and it was her wicked sense of humor that got us through the wacky faux paus. Jillian is pee-your-pants funny. She does a hilarious Picasso skit of me that has the entire crew crying from laughing so hard.

For Jillian, it was an easy transition, but not so much for others. One celebrity I worked with said she loved her makeup, but when she found out what products I used, she asked me to replace them all with name brands. It was disheartening. She liked the way she looked—my technique, color choices, and design—but she still wanted premium makeup. When you can afford the gold standard, that's what you want . . . at least until you know better. It didn't matter to her that it was healthier or that it worked as well. She wanted premium and she got it! End. Of. Story.

I understand this desire for premium products wholeheartedly. I like quality. I want everything I touch to be a magical experience. I want a beautiful presentation. I want my products to look pretty, feel luxurious, and smell fabulous. I want to have an outer body experience when I hold them. And I am like that with everything—food, clothes, interior design, entertainment—you name it. I want to be enchanted. I have been this way since I was a child, poring over the glossy pages of fashion and lifestyle magazines, envisioning a life that only existed in my dreams.

My clients weren't the only challenge either. Beauty editors, experts, and even friends said I couldn't create pretty faces with chemically safe cosmetics. They weren't trying to be negative or unsupportive; they simply didn't want me to fail. They didn't have the vision that I had. I could see the movement toward natural cosmetics happening already, and I knew I could figure out how to successfully transition my professional makeup kits to chemically safe cosmetics.

MY LEARNING CURVE

Having decided to continue on my eco-path, the learning curve was massive. I remember calling all of the green beauty companies at the time and asking them to send me products. I tested and continue to test many products. I would sit on the living room floor, mirror in hand, products fanned out in front of me. So many of them didn't perform. The colors were insipid and muddy, the texture too greasy or grabby, the smell was either off, or there was no scent at all. Understandably, the packaging was not pretty. Small companies didn't have money to put into packaging, so I overlooked that, but the formula had to work.

I gave products to friends to try, too, and surveyed them on their thoughts, which were most often unfavorable reviews. Time and time again I heard the same things: "I am really into smell" or "I like nice packaging," or "Chanel has a product like it that's much better." I knew what they were going to say before they said it. But I wanted to know what they liked about it, if anything, and how they used it.

What I found was that with the early green products, you really had to work them and know how to work *with* them, add to them, or layer them. To get the look of a Nars Orgasm Blush, you had to use two or three products. I was fine with that as long as I knew how to achieve the look. My fussy friends, however, were not. And who could blame them? Now you can find chemically safe blush that looks like Nars Orgasm. It's called Zuii Organic Certified Organic Flora Blush in Melon. You don't have to layer several colors to achieve the look like I had to a decade ago.

If a product was ambiguous, I called the company saying, "Your face wash lists fragrance in the ingredients and it doesn't say from essential oils or anything about it being a natural fragrance or blend, but your packaging says 'all natural.' What is this fragrance made of?"

They would always tell me the truth. Sometimes it was essential oils or a blend, other times it was synthetic. You often have to call and ask.

Being so green (no pun intended), I wasn't able to figure out true-blue chemically safe products or companies. It's hard to know from the packaging. They are tricky, and I didn't know anything about government regulations (or lack thereof) at the time. Simply put, I couldn't identify "green washing" so easily: companies that make you think they are eco-friendly and/or chemically safe but really aren't. These are companies that used the word "natural" and put flowers on their packaging but filled their product with 99 percent synthetics and only 1 percent botanicals. Then there were the companies that removed some of the major offenders but not all. Some just took out the buzzword chemicals, like parabens and sodium lauryl (or laureth) sulfate. Honestly, at the time, I was happy with the ones that just took out some of the major offenders, because I still needed the product to do my job, and it gave me more options for color when I needed it. To this day I will still use a traditional lipstick if I need a certain color option. For example, you can't find a natural florescent pink lipstick. It doesn't exist. I'll tell you why I am okay with that in Chapter 5. There is a place and a time for it.

Along the way, I've read green blogs, written green blogs on my website (*PaigePadgett.com*), gone to lectures when I could find them, and in general immersed myself in anything about toxic chemicals in makeup. The Environmental Working Group (*EWG; www.ewg .org*) proved to be the best source of information, along with the Campaign for Safe Cosmetics (*www.safecosmetics.org*) and Women's Voices for the Earth (*www.womensvoices.org*). I consult them religiously even now.

Then, finally, in 2006, when no one else had done it, I successfully greened my professional kit. I was a green beauty pioneer.

WHAT IS GREEN?

L et me be very clear here. This book is not written for the purists. It's for the average woman who cares about style and luxury, and loves cosmetics above all. It is intended to help you rid toxic chemicals from your body or at best offset some of your body burden. It's not meant to be rigidly chemically free or restrictive. It is meant to be easily incorporated and inclusive rather than exclusive of products that make you happy and confident.

For the purpose of this book, green cosmetics are defined as formulated to be nontoxic to humans and the environment. These are products that are made without harmful chemicals, including but not limited to parabens, synthetic fragrances, dyes, and sulfates. Some of these same products are USDA Organic, ECOCERT, or hold seals from other eco-friendly certifying bodies. Green or chemically safe products are not necessarily 100 percent natural. Not all chemicals are toxic. The EWG regards some chemicals as being relatively harmless to the body.

> If you only wanted to use 100 percent organic makeup, you'd never have a full face of makeup—ever.

Green beauty isn't always organic either. In general, organic makeup is difficult to formulate. And while much of the mineral-based cosmetics contain organic ingredients, minerals can't be certified organic. That's why you won't find certified organic makeup but you will find skin care and other products that don't use colorants or minerals. If you only wanted to use 100 percent organic makeup, you'd never have a full face of makeup—ever.

Green terminology can be misleading. For me, being green means that a product is chemically safe and eco-friendly. However, it does not necessarily mean that it's all natural or organic; that's a bonus. I will use the terms "green,""chemically safe,""eco-friendly," and "natural" interchangeably.

I am against animal testing or animal cruelty of any kind. For most manufacturers, "cruelty-free" has nothing to do with producing green products. Traditional cosmetic companies can be cruelty-free, so beware of the cruelty-free labeling—it does not mean the product is natural or chemically safe. I maintain a high standard for green makeup and do not consider a product eco-friendly if it is not cruelty-free. In *The Green Beauty Rules*, my eco-friendly product recommendations are formulated cruelty-free.

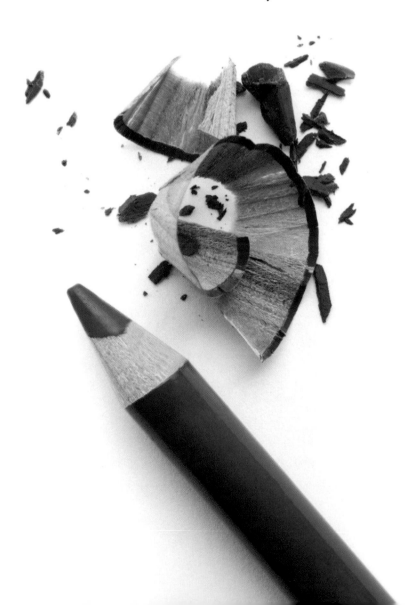

The Five
Green Beauty Myths

Over the years, I've heard all the misconceptions and reasons why women don't or won't try to use green cosmetics. Let's take a look at the five biggest green myths:

MYTH #1: GREEN PRODUCTS COST TOO MUCH. Green products are not necessarily more expensive. Like traditional products, you'll find a wide range from drugstore and mass-marketed to luxury brands. For example, you can find chemically safe shampoo from $9 to $35. However, similar to food, you will often pay more for organic products. Like anything, the higher the quality of the product, the more you will pay for it. If a product is certified from an organization like the USDA or ECOCERT (which we'll learn more about in Chapter 3), it may be costlier but not always. Organic Wear by Physicians Formula is extremely affordable, and many (not all) of the products are ECOCERT. Products that include descriptions such as "biodynamic," "wild-crafted," "fair trade," "organic," or "cold-pressed" in the ingredients list may cost more but are worth it in the long run. It's really up to you. The question is, what do you want and how much are you willing to pay for it?

MYTH #2: IT'S TOO TIME-CONSUMING TO FIND GREEN PRODUCTS. Once you know what you are doing, it doesn't take more time to find (or use) green products. There is a learning curve to understanding toxic chemicals and how to eliminate them, but that's where I come in. Hopefully this book will make that curve much smaller for you. Once you've learned how to green your beauty routine, you will spend the same amount of time shopping for chemically safe cosmetics and applying them as you would for any of your traditional products.

MYTH #3: GREEN PRODUCTS SACRIFICE QUALITY. Green products do work. There is no denying that traditional products produce amazing results and that sometimes chemically safe options won't compare to the traditional formulas. Let's get that out of the way right now. It's about your commitment and knowing how and when to use a traditional product. However, natural ingredients have become highly sophisticated. There are quality nontoxic replacements for just about every toxic petrochemical. White willow bark and grape seed extract, for example, can be used instead of parabens. Colors are more vibrant now with the use of flowers. Natural and chemically safe alternatives for silicone in hair care and skin care products are available. In Chapter 7, I will list my favorite products so it will take all the guesswork out of it for you.

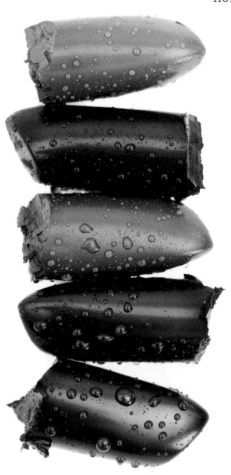

MYTH #4: GREEN PRODUCTS LACK GLAMOUR. You don't have to sacrifice glamour. Think about all the supermodels and actresses who have eco-friendly-marketed product lines. Victoria's Secret model Miranda Kerr founded a natural bath and body line called KORA. Josie Maran, the face of Maybelline for years, launched an eco-conscious makeup line in her name. Supermodel Gisele Bündchen created Sejaa, a 100 percent natural spa skin care line. It doesn't get any sexier than that. In addition, there are thousands of chemically safe products on the market that are glamorous, with beautiful packaging, excellent branding, and premium ingredients. If you want high-end products, you can have them. Don't you want a body lotion made with the finest oils from all over the globe? That's glamorous!

MYTH #5: IT'S INCONVENIENT TO FIND GREEN PRODUCTS. Green products are easier than ever to find. You can find them just about anywhere, even at the airport, which is important to me. There are a myriad of mass cosmetic lines sold in drugstores (see the sidebar Drugstore Superstars in Chapter 6) and box stores like Walgreens, CVS, Target, and Walmart. You can also conveniently find them online at a variety of boutique green stores and larger e-commerce sites such as amazon.com and drugstore.com. You don't have to hunt them down like you used to. In Chapter 6, I'll tell you where I like to shop.

Boom! The biggest green beauty myths are busted.

Now it's your turn to be a green beauty pioneer. As you begin to think about your own beauty journey, who are your inspirations? Who do you admire? Do you prefer a light touch, glowing skin, or accentuated, arched brows? Do you treat makeup as a luxury, reveling in the process of making up your face? Or are you more minimal, keeping it simple and carefree? Really think about where your view of beauty and makeup came from and how you've nurtured this part of your life. If we were to open your cosmetic bag today, what would it say about you—and would you like what it said?

YOUR TURN

Think about your attachment to your products. Are you fearful of parting ways with some of your longtime favorites? Is it the significance of the brand? Is it the performance, the reliability, or just the look you've taken years to perfect? How attached are you to the look, smell, or even the touch of your favorite face cream or lipstick? Maybe a particular brand of blush reminds you of a happy time in your life.

Or makeup could be a hobby for you. Are all of your magazines dog-eared to the latest trends and must-haves in beauty? Do you love spending a Saturday afternoon browsing and experimenting in Sephora? Are you a product junkie or do you consider a new cosmetic a splurge, saving until you can buy that premium brand?

I work in the beauty industry, and it is driven by fashion. I am also a true consumer. I shop in stores and online for products. Sure, I will make the occasional lip scrub or hair mask at home, but I'm no Betty Crocker of beauty. What's more, I don't want to be. So the green-cosmetics-not-being-seen-as-chic dilemma has not escaped me. But rather than reject what I know to be true, I have chosen to embrace it and change the stereotype and stigma of eco-friendly cosmetics.

Why are you interested in green beauty? What is your motivation? Are you already living clean in other areas of your life so this is the natural next step? Are you excited about making this transformation? Maybe this is the first step for you, and it's easier to focus on what you put on your body rather than what you put into it. Ah, but it's a slippery slope. In no time at all you will be shooting shots of turmeric and wheat grass. Ha! But really, think about what is pushing you toward this change. Is it for you, your family, your future, or our planet?

For me, there were a few ah-ha moments that spurred me along, but the biggest factor by far was that I wanted to be healthy and alive for a very long time. I wanted to make sure I was doing the things that would keep me around to see my daughter grow up, even though I didn't have her at the time I knew I would. I was already in my late thirties, and I knew I was going to be an older mom. Now at the age of forty-seven, I want to make sure I am not only alive but that I am healthy enough to enjoy life with my daughter. I realize there are no guarantees in life and in health, but I want to feel good about my decisions. This is perhaps the single most important reason I choose to green my beauty routine. But it's not only that I want to be healthy; I also don't want to leave a legacy of an unhealthy earth. I want to leave a clean, healthy earth for our children, grandchildren, and future generations. For me there is a micro-element (personal) and a macro-element (global) to my approach to a green lifestyle and green beauty.

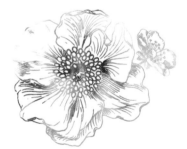

YOUR ECO-ATTITUDE:
THREE LEVELS OF SUSTAINABILITY

I have created three levels of sustainability when it comes to greening your beauty routine. I call them eco-attitudes. The idea is that if you start at the most elementary level, "Green Beauty Beginner," with time you will move into "Green Beauty Pro" and perhaps even "Green Beauty Master." I believe in giving women choices and taking baby steps. Making the switch from your favorite products and premium brands takes time. There is a mental shift that needs to take place, and there is a learning curve, too. You won't go from using Armani and Dior to using Jane Iredale and ZuZu Luxe in one day. Not that you can't—you can—but everyone works at a different pace. Some people are all-in right away while others need a little more time to transition. No judgment here!

Listed below are three different eco-attitudes. Choose the description that you most relate to now, depending on your season of life and your surrounding circumstances. These commitment levels should serve as a starting point and a guide. You'll either bounce between eco-attitudes (I do) or commit wholeheartedly to one. The hope is that you'll advance through each level and beyond. This book will jump-start your transition to clean. I want you to take in the information and run with it.

Which best describes your eco-attitude?

GREEN BEAUTY BEGINNER: You are just being introduced to chemically safe cosmetics and go for the green products that have removed some of the major offenders. Your eco-efforts include reusing your shopping bags, drinking out of a SIGG bottle, and ordering fair-trade coffee. At the end of the day, you want to reduce your cosmetic footprint but can't live without your signature scent.

GREEN BEAUTY PRO: You are well versed in green cosmetics and enjoy trying a variety of green products that are chemically safe, natural, and organic. You are highly concerned about the welfare of the earth. You make sacrifices and are committed to better health. You can't imagine not helping to maintain a healthy planet. You drive a hybrid or other low emissions vehicle and only buy organic produce from the local farmer's market. You refuse to drink bottled water and yet you don't get your knickers in a twist if others around you do.

GREEN BEAUTY MASTER: You have a deep knowledge of toxic chemicals in cosmetics and the environment and seek out only the purest products often with few ingredients. You passionately advocate for the health of our planet and reuse, reduce, and recycle with zeal. No expense was spared when you installed your gray-water system in your solar-powered home. You're committed to creating awareness about our planet's resources and are involved in your community to inspire others to make the same efforts as you.

Are you pleased with your eco-attitude? You will be referring back to it in Chapter 6. Remember, there is no wrong or right commitment level. It's what you can handle at the time that will best support your long-term success. I have found that an eco-attitude is a mind-set that can last anywhere from a moment to a decade. You'll see. The deeper you get into the process, the more you will find your actions toward greening will become second nature.

Bounce between the three eco-attitudes if you feel like it, and you probably will. I certainly do. There are occasions when I feel I need a particular product in my life, whether it's a body bronzer by a company that has only taken out the major chemical offenders or a lipstick that I love for its color, or when I am traveling and am forced to shop for toiletries in airports. Sometimes I find superclean products and sometimes I don't. After my twenty-six-hour flight to India, I am a little less discriminating when considering my options. Sometimes you have to make do with what you have. At the very least, I can usually find a product or two in any airport or drugstore that is absent of parabens and a few synthetics.

There are the rare times, usually for work, that I grab a particular product because I need something I know works, without trial and error. You can't age someone by thirty years or turn them blue without some chemicals. Not yet anyway. I don't want to hold up production or upset the photographer because my product isn't working properly. You may be a sleep-deprived new mom or busy college student with limited time and money. There are many reasons you may choose to use a product that is not as clean as you prefer. Don't worry—I'm going to teach you how to balance it all out. No matter where you start, you will build the confidence and skill to move on to the next category. The progression is the natural course of greening. I love to have choices, don't you? The good thing is that with this book as your guide, you can.

I want to be honest with you. I am a work in progress too. I don't know everything there is to know about chemicals and cosmetics, and I strive to find a balance between living clean and living stylishly. While my beauty routines are 90 percent clean most of the time, I know I have room for improvement and refinement. It has taken me years to gain my knowledge and I learn something new daily, whether it's about a toxic chemical, how two chemicals react together, or another name for a toxic chemical. I have discovered a slew of alternatives for preservatives, chemical exfoliators, and even Botox! It's a whole new world. I am constantly rethinking and reevaluating my position on certain chemicals, but my philosophy remains the same: *Beauty doesn't have to be toxic. Be clean when you can and where it counts.*

Think about the reason you want to green your beauty routine. Jillian Michaels asks people to define their "why" when thinking of reasons they want to get healthy. This is because you must be able to articulate a meaningful reason for creating change. The decision to make the change happens in your heart, not your head. What we care about most will drive our behavior. It's the same for greening your beauty routine.

Why do you want to detoxify your beauty routine? Do you have allergies or sensitivities? Is it to be around for your children or spouse? Is it to travel or dance longer? Is it to have a healthy baby? What does it look like in your life?

This process isn't just about making over your products; it's also about creating the vision of who you want to be, so that as you green your routine, you'll know exactly what you need to do to support it. My hope for you is that over the course of our time together, you will take what you learn, implement it in your own life, and share it with those who matter to you.

Chapter Two

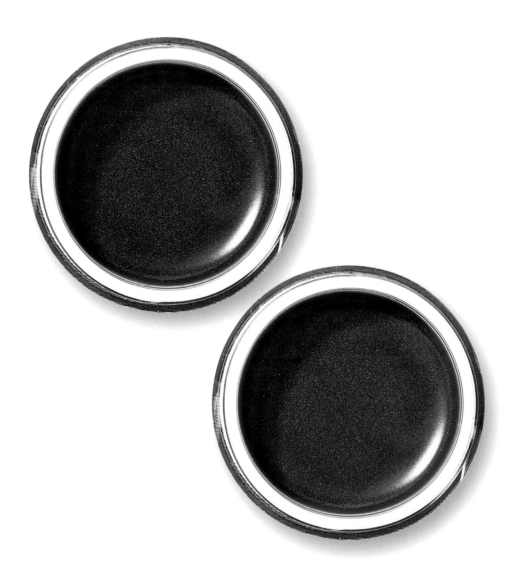

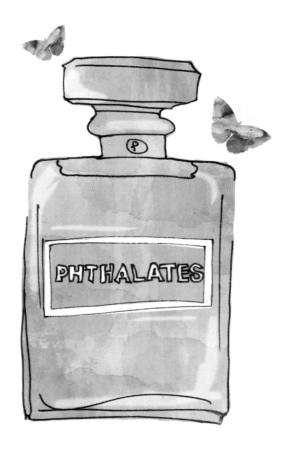

BEAUTY from the
"Outside In"

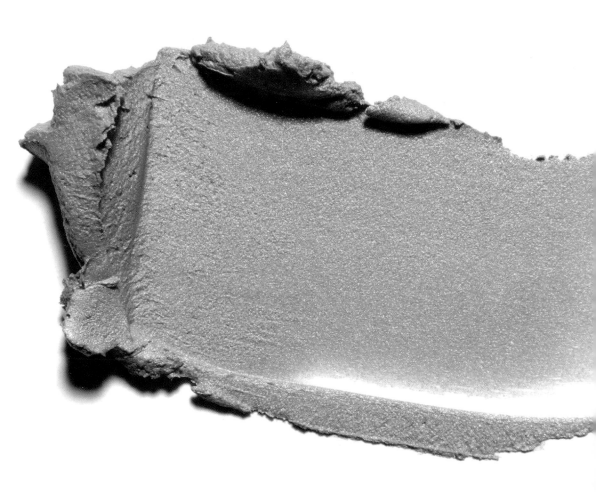

I consider what I put *on* my body equally as important as what I put *in* it. My beauty diet is a highly integral part of my overall health, and I credit Ken Cook, founder of the Environmental Working Group (EWG), for the shift in my perspective.

One evening many years ago I attended his lecture "Ten Americans," where he spoke about the far-reaching effects of toxicity (you can view the lecture on the EWG website at http://www.ewg.org/news/videos/10-americans). Ken explained how the American Red Cross took a random sampling of blood from ten Americans across the United States. The blood was then examined by researchers from two objective, major laboratories. Every American sampled had an average of 287 toxic chemicals in their system. The sources of the chemicals were from a variety of categories, including industrial, pesticides, pharmaceutical, and household. Large portions of the toxic chemicals were also from cosmetics. The most astounding aspect of this sampling is that none of the Americans tested had ever worked in a factory or field, applied cosmetics of any kind, or had ever cleaned a home. The testing population was fetuses, and the blood samples had been taken from umbilical cords. Our babies were being born with Viagra and Paxil in their bodies. This was shocking!

Here are some statistics from the talk: the blood was sampled for 413 toxic chemicals. Approximately 287 industrial chemicals were detected in the blood samples. An average of 200 industrial chemicals and pollutants were found per baby. Of the average 287 chemicals detected in the umbilical cord blood:

- 134 cause cancer.

- 130 cause immune system toxicity.

- 158 are neurotoxins.

- 186 cause infertility.

- 151 cause birth defects.

- 154 cause hormone disruption.

- 186 cause infertility.

- 212 are industrial chemicals and pesticides that were banned more than thirty years ago.

- 28 are waste byproducts.

- 47 are consumer product ingredients.

- 168 were from 12 personal care products that women use daily.

- 85 were from ingredients from 6 personal care products that men use daily.

In addition, while a portion of what we put on our bodies stays in our bodies, the remaining chemicals make their way into our disposal systems. Chemicals end up in our water supply, our crops and livestock, and back into our bodies. These harmful cosmetic chemicals that reenter the environment are defined by the Environmental Protection Agency (EPA) as PPCPs: Pharmaceuticals and Personal Care Products. As pollutants, PPCPs refer to any product used by individuals for personal health or cosmetic reasons or used by agribusiness to enhance the growth or health of livestock. PPCPs comprise a diverse collection of thousands of chemical substances, including prescription and over-the-counter (OTC) therapeutic drugs, veterinary drugs, fragrances, and cosmetics.

The EPA estimates that more than three million tons of personal care chemicals are dumped into waterways each year, adversely impacting our ecosystem. When we shower or bathe, everything we use on our bodies goes down the drain—from shampoo, soap, body lotions, perfumes, hair dye, face wash, glycolic acids, and other corrosive skin care products. Pretty much anything you use goes into the waterway, and these toxic chemicals are being recycled right into our food supplies. What's more, the packaging and disposal of these products negatively affects our environment when they end up in landfills and leach into the earth. This is how our planet is a closed circuit. Nothing escapes it. It's all simply recycled in one way or another.

Ken's talk blew me away. I decided that I would learn how to eliminate toxic chemicals from my cosmetics and teach others how to do it as well. It was one of those moments when you feel like you've found the missing piece of the puzzle. His inspiration gave me the greater sense of purpose that I had been seeking in my career as a makeup artist. From that day forward, I was fully committed to a green beauty lifestyle, not just for myself but for others as well.

YOUR BEAUTY ROUTINE IS A DIET

Your skin literally eats your beauty products. Cosmetic products act like food for your skin, and chemicals end up in your pores and in your bloodstream, traveling throughout your body. It's called transdermal delivery. Skin is the largest organ of the body; it lives and breathes. The skin acts as a barrier, preventing germs and toxins from getting into the body and preventing water and moisture from escaping the body. However, it's not a complete barrier, and your body *can* take in toxins, vitamins and minerals, medicine, and other chemicals. In fact, the skin absorbs 60 percent of what you put on it. It is considered a "major entry route" into the body. The World Health Organization supports this statement in a report published in 2005.[1]

The problem with traditional cosmetics is that the bad stuff comes with the good stuff. And since skin is the largest organ of the body, it can potentially take in large amounts of toxins. Even in low dosages, chemicals are sometimes bioaccumulative, meaning the chemicals never leave our system and accumulate in the body over decades.

Cosmetic products are like food in that they ultimately get metabolized by the body. Because of this fact, transdermal delivery is most often used as a highly effective medicinal treatment method. It's not new; for thousands of years, people have placed substances on the skin for therapeutic effects. It's most common uses today are for pain management, birth control, and smoking cessation. The following explains how transdermal delivery works.

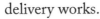

SKIN ABSORPTION

I f the molecular weight of a substance is small enough to pass through your skin, it will end up in your body. Whether it's in a spray, soak, gel, lotion, or cream, it will enter your body if it is small enough. What's more, this major route of entry bypasses the liver and kidneys, entering the bloodstream directly without having the added protection of filtering out toxins from the liver and being flushed away by the kidneys. One fun way for you to see for yourself how transdermal absorption works is to rub a garlic clove on the bottom of your bare foot and smell your breath thirty minutes later. You will be surprised that you can smell the garlic.

Consider this warning from the EWG: "Cosmetic ingredients do not remain on the surface of the skin. They are designed to penetrate, and they do. Scientists have found many common cosmetic ingredients in human tissues, including phthalates in urine, preservatives called parabens in breast tumor tissue, and persistent fragrance components in human fat. Do the concentrations at which they are typically found pose risks? For the most part, those studies have not been done. But a small but growing number of studies serve as scientific red flags."[2]

Everyone varies in the amount of substance they absorb through the skin. Hair follicles, sweat ducts, skin thickness, and barrier accessibility are some of the factors that control how the skin will absorb a substance. However, there are some ways we can control how much of a substance is absorbed into the body. This is important, because you can use it to your advantage in keeping toxins out and allowing the good stuff in. Here are some ways to control the delivery of a substance transdermally.

FIVE WAYS TO CONTROL TRANSDERMAL ABSORPTION

1. **AREA SIZE:** Increasing the area of skin you are applying the substance to increases absorption. The larger the body area of application, the more your body will absorb. For example, a body lotion will deliver more of its ingredients than a face cream.

2. **DURATION/FREQUENCY:** Penetration occurs over time. The longer you leave it on, the more you will absorb. Increasing the frequency of application will also allow the skin to absorb more product.

3. **LOCATION:** Absorption rates will vary in different parts of the body. Certain areas of the body, like the soles of the feet, forehead, and scalp take in more of the substance.

4. **AMOUNT:** Applying more of a substance increases the amount absorbed. Penetration will stop usually when the skin is saturated.

5. **HYDRATION:** Well-hydrated skin is easier to penetrate than dry skin.

Keep these points in mind when choosing to use a product that is not chemically safe. Where are you applying the product? How large is the area? For how long are you applying it? For example, if you cannot live without your favorite body bronzer or hydrator and it's not chemically safe, you will be absorbing the toxins more than pretty much any other product you use since it is being used on the entire body.

USE IT TO YOUR ADVANTAGE

N ow that you know the negative effects of transdermal delivery, there are three ways to make it work for you.

1. **HYDRATE WHEN USING CHEMICALLY SAFE PRODUCTS.**
   For example, if you have sore muscles, try soaking in a hot bath with Dead Sea salt and essential oils. I love baths. The magnesium in the salt relaxes the muscles and flushes out the lactic acid. For enhanced benefits, I add essential oils, milk, or clay. Also, when applying a chemically safe face cream, mist your face first before moisturizing. The water helps the cream penetrate the skin.

2. **USE NUTRIENT RICH PRODUCTS.** I know that when I apply makeup, body products, or hair care, my body is getting quality ingredients that nourish the skin instead of poison it.

3. **USE PRODUCTS THAT OFFER EXTRA BENEFITS, SUCH AS VITAMINS, ANTIOXIDANTS, AND BOTANICAL EXTRACTS.**
   If you're going to be absorbing product, try to use products with health-promoting ingredients, like antioxidants. Antioxidants inhibit free-radical damage and do the job of reducing environmental damage whether it is from the sun, pollution, or just the very air we breathe.

This book is about beauty. My goal here is to keep you as radiant as you already are and then amplify that with an overall feeling of well-being and satisfaction through healthy decisions with your cosmetics. Beauty always starts from the inside out, and you may already be doing everything within your power to nurture your body, mind, and soul. But what you put *on* your body is as important as what you put *into* it.

THE 80/20 RULE

E ven with a strict nutritional diet, everyone needs a cheat day or a favorite cheat food. Ice cream anyone? That's my kryptonite. It makes dieting easier and more enjoyable, and you are more likely to stick to it. Your beauty diet is no different. I have found the best way to do this is to use the 80/20 rule—80 percent of your beauty routine should be clean while 20 percent can be comprised of your favorite things that may contain "the nasties." (You'll learn more about the nasties in Chapter 4.)

One way you can determine your 20 percent is to calculate the products you use in your daily grooming routine. If you use ten products daily, at least eight should be chemically safe. It's a bit simplified, but it's a good starting point. I'd rather you start greening your routine straightaway rather than become bogged down with the mathematical ratio. It's difficult to determine exactly 20 percent. You have to make your best judgment.

I strive to keep my routine 100 percent chemically safe, but in reality, it's about 90 percent chemically safe after factoring in a few things I choose to keep. Some products alone could easily measure 20 percent, because they have so many toxic chemicals in them. Fragrance is one example. I adore fragrance. It's my ice-cream sundae. It enhances my mood and lifts my spirit, evoking a kind of nostalgia that makes me feel really happy and energized. Putting all these great things aside, the reality is that the very nature of fragrance is petrochemicals. With that in mind, I am careful to use it as my 20 percent and exercise caution of use by spraying it on my clothes and hair, to avoid direct contact with my skin. Sometimes I spray it in the air and walk through it, which gives me a pleasant undertone of scent. When I do this, I cover my face and I try not to breathe it in. You don't want it in your lungs any more than on your skin or in your bloodstream. I understand that chemicals on clothes can leach into your body as well, and the smell of perfume can cause allergies and sinus irritation among other things, but not to the degree as if directly applied to your skin or if you inhaled the perfume itself. Limiting exposure by using fragrance less or indirectly as I do is a good way to reduce your exposure to chemicals.

Only you know what you can and cannot allow for. Everyone will have different criteria and desires. I want to highlight how you can allow for chemicals and measure (to some degree) your chemical allowance. Here are three easy ways you can calculate your 20 percent toxic chemical allowance. You will find they are similar to the principals listed above for skin absorption.

1. **CALCULATE:** Add up your daily products and allow 20 percent for your favorite must-have traditional products. If you use ten products, eight should be clean and two can be cheat products. This is the easiest way to calculate, but it's a very loose method to determine your 20 percent, as it doesn't factor in the toxicity of the ingredients in each product.

2. **FREQUENCY:** Use your highly toxic cheat products only once a month or once a week if you must. That is what I do with my favorite fragrances, as I mentioned earlier.

3. **APPLICATION:** Apply less of a cheat product when you do use it and apply it to a smaller area if possible.

Employ the knowledge you now have about skin absorption and transdermal delivery. Knowledge is going to be your best defense for your chemical allowance. The more you know, the easier it will be to determine how to use your 20 percent chemical allowance. Once you have read this book, it will be easy for you to determine when, where, and how to use your cheat products. With this knowledge comes intuition. Let your intuition guide you. Trust yourself. You can do this.

How are you feeling? I know it's a lot to take in, but we're baby stepping in stilettos, so it's all worth it, right? Next, we launch into what "natural," "organic," and "naturally derived" really mean, as well as reading labels; making sense of all the certifications, seals, and stamps; and identifying toxic chemicals.

Nine No-Brainer Tips to Green Your Beauty Routine

1. **DON'T FEEL OVERWHELMED.** Start slowly; you don't have to buy everything at once.

2. **STOP USING DISPOSABLES.** Use washcloths instead of makeup wipes, use a reusable sponge, and get a real razor.

3. **USE EVERY LAST DROP OF** your lip gloss, every fleck of eye shadow, and sharpen your pencils until they are nubs before you replace them.

4. **USE FEWER PRODUCTS AND LESS OF THEM.**

5. **BUY PRODUCTS THAT MULTITASK:** for example, body balms, BB creams, and multisticks.

6. **SEEK OUT PRODUCTS/COMPANIES** that use minimal packaging.

7. **RECYCLE** when you can.

8. **FIX BROKEN PRESSED POWDERS.** Yes. (see DIY page 90).

9. **REMEMBER, IT'S NOT ALL OR NOTHING.** Go at your own pace.

Chapter Three

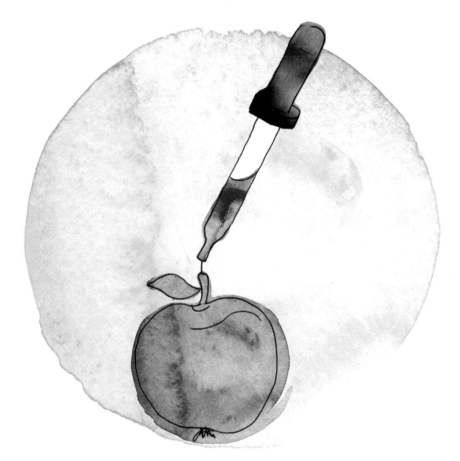

ORGANIC, Natural, and Naturally *Derived*

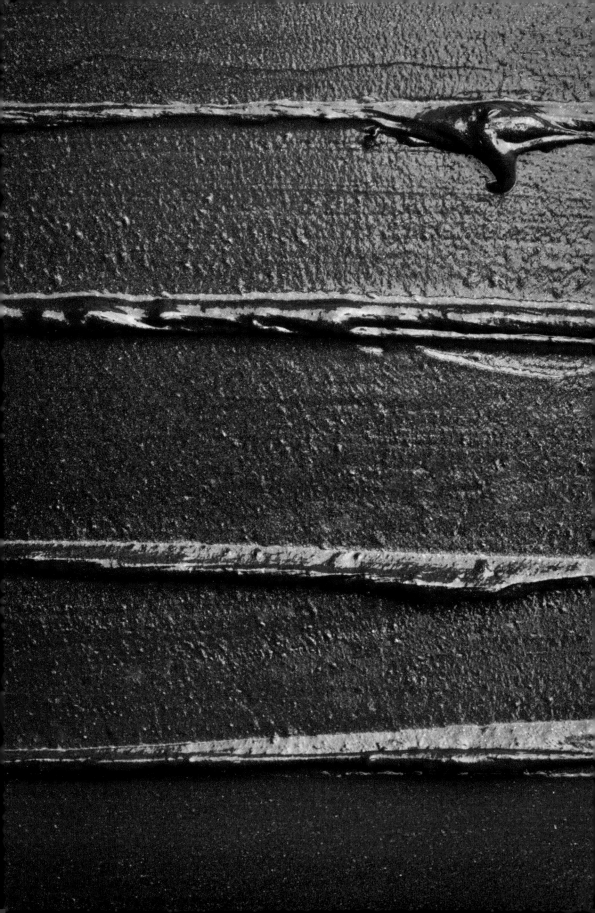

In today's cosmetics market, you may think you need a chemistry degree to decode the natural cosmetic jargon. The terms are often used improperly or they can be used to obscure and "greenwash" (according to *Merriam Webster's Collegiate Dictionary,* "greenwashing" involves "expressions of environmentalist concerns, especially as a cover for products, policies, or activities"). Some companies advertise products as "natural" or "organic" to give the impression that they are green when indeed they are not. This greenwashing causes confusion and often results in the consumer not knowing what to believe.

It's a typical scenario. You go to the drugstore looking for a natural product. To your delight, you find an entire aisle of shelves stocked with natural-looking products. You grab the pretty bottle (that's my inclination too) with botanical imagery and earthy serene colors on the packaging. The word "natural" is printed on the packaging. Being the savvy shopper you are, you check the ingredients, hoping to see it chock-full of healthy, nourishing stuff only to see a few recognizable ingredients on the label, which sadly include fragrance and parabens. You feel your excitement melt away as disappointment and frustration take over.

When I first began my green beauty journey and started seeking out chemically safe and natural products, I checked out hundreds of products posing as natural or organic only to find that there were merely a few natural or organic ingredients among a load of petrochemicals. It was disheartening.

Several years back, while shopping for a shoot at one of my favorite beauty supply stores in the San Fernando Valley, I was hoping to find fabulous, chemically safe makeup alternatives to use on my client. I was thrilled to find one mineral line, a kitschy boutique brand that was fun and edgy. I filled my basket with lipsticks, eye shadows, and blush in the most amazing colors. Then, just before checking out, I gave the ingredient list a quick look to make sure they were as clean as they claimed. I was crushed. The products were filled with parabens and petrochemicals. I had to put all the products back. I never made that mistake again! I became a box turner straightaway. Now I temper my enthusiasm until after I check the ingredient labels. A decade ago we didn't have the options we do today. Even the larger companies who championed environmental causes and sustainability, like Aveda and the Body Shop, didn't have chemically safe formulations when I greened my beauty kits in 2006. I was a huge fan of both companies for their environmental, animal and human rights efforts but I couldn't use the cosmetics. I admired Horst Rechelbacher, Aveda founder, and Anita Roddick, The Body Shop founder, for their great environmental activism. Legend has it Horst once drank an Aveda hairspray to demonstrate how clean it was. It was heart breaking to me because I grew up with Aveda products and loved them, but by 2006 Aveda had long been sold to Estée Lauder and the formulas contained parabens and synthetic dyes.

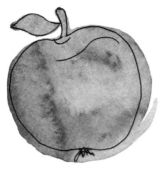

Cosmetic Chemistry Decoded

COSMETIC: The Federal Food, Drug, and Cosmetic Act (FD&C Act) defines cosmetics as "articles intended to be rubbed, poured, sprinkled, or sprayed on, introduced into, or otherwise applied to the human body . . . for cleansing, beautifying, promoting attractiveness, or altering the appearance; a product used for beautification or hygiene."

NATURAL: According to the National Organics Program (NOP), a natural substance is derived from a plant, mineral, or animal source, without having undergone a synthetic process. Physical and biological processes can still render a substance as natural.

ORGANIC: The USDA defines organic as follows: "Organic agriculture is an ecological production management system that promotes and enhances biodiversity, biological cycles, and soil biological activity. It is based on minimal use of off-farm inputs and on management practices that restore, maintain, and enhance ecological harmony."

BIODYNAMIC: refers to a process that is more holistic than organic in farming and food production. The same rules apply as organic processes, but farmers also strive to achieve harmony with the earth through weather and climate patterns that work together to create balance.

NATURALLY DERIVED: refers to materials where the majority of the molecular structure (not less than 50 percent by weight) is derived from natural materials as defined above.

NATURE IDENTICAL: substances that exist in nature but are produced in a lab.

NONSYNTHETIC: same as natural.

SYNTHETIC: The NOP definition of a synthetic is a substance that has been formulated or manufactured by a chemical process, and has chemically altered a substance that was derived from a naturally occurring plant, mineral, or animal source.

SUSTAINABILITY: refers to the endurance of eco-systems and processes; the biological ability to remain diverse and productive; the ability to be sustained, supported, upheld as relating to the method of harvest or using natural resources; able to be maintained or sustained at a certain level or rate.

CRUELTY-FREE: products have not been tested on animals or have been manufactured or developed by methods that do not experiment on, harm, or kill animals.

VEGAN: rejects the use of animals and cruelty to animals for food, clothing, and other purposes; items that are free of animal byproducts; one who does not eat or use materials that come from animals.

NATURAL AND ORGANIC

Do you reach for products that say the words natural and organic in hopes of purchasing a pure product? If so, you will be disappointed to know a product isn't clean just because it says it's natural or organic. It's easy to be fooled. Packaging and marketing can look highly convincing. The words "natural" and "organic" are not regulated by the FDA for use on personal care products because the terms have no definition under the FD&C Act, which is the law that defines how cosmetics are regulated. Similarly, the European Union has no definition for natural or organic cosmetics. The term "natural" is not regulated at all, so it means absolutely nothing. What's more, it means different things to different people. Most products contain some natural ingredients, but that doesn't mean they are all natural or even chemically safe.

Likewise, simply because a product says it's organic doesn't mean it is. It may have some organic ingredients but that doesn't mean the entire product is organic. What's in the other ingredients? Does it contain synthetic preservatives, fragrances, or dyes? Many personal care products use the term "organic" on their label, packaging, or in their name. Because of the lax regulation of the term, this is not prohibited. Only when a product is certified by the USDA National Organic Program does the term have some regulation. Cosmetics that are USDA Organic are certified according to USDA food standards, which exclusively apply to ingredients that are grown. It's an excellent standard and a seal that can you can trust. The guidelines are straightforward, so it's easy to understand and you know what you're getting when you see the stamp. I consider it a very good seal to look for when shopping.

> Simply because a product says it's organic doesn't mean it is.

Seals are important on packaging because they show that a product has undergone a third-party review process as opposed to a normal, conventional product that doesn't have the seal. The claims and ingredients have been reviewed by a company other than the one that is marketing the product. Seals maintain a standard for natural and organic cosmetics that promotes ingredients from renewable resources, requires specific minimum levels of organic content in the products, and provides an environmentally friendly product in itself.

THE USDA NATIONAL ORGANIC PROGRAM SEAL OF APPROVAL

In order for a product to use the term "100 percent organic," it must be just that—excluding water and salt. All ingredients must be organic. To use the USDA Organic seal, a product must be at least "95 percent organic," excluding water and salt. To use the term "organic," a product must contain 70 percent or more organic ingredients. If a product has less than 70 percent organic ingredients, the term "organic" is not allowed on the label anywhere.

In addition to the USDA Organic seal, there are a variety of governmental, independent, domestic, and international certification programs to help consumers feel more confident that they are getting quality natural cosmetics (see the sidebar Natural and Organic Cosmetic Seals). Choosing a product with a reputable certification is one way I know I am getting a clean product.

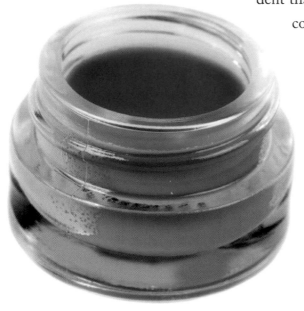

Natural and Organic Cosmetic Seals

AGRICULTURE BIOLOGIQUE—EU: "Organic" label: at least 95 percent organic.

AUSTRALIAN CERTIFIED ORGANIC: "Organic" label: at least 95 percent organic.

BDIH—GERMANY: Complies with COSMetic Organic Standard (COSMOS; COSMOS was developed as a private standard by five charter members: BDIH [Germany], Cosmebio [France], Ecocert Greenlife SAS [France], ICEA [Italy], and the Soil Association [Great Britain]).

BIO—GERMANY: "Bio" label: at least 95 percent organic.

CAAQ—CANADA: "Made with organic": at least 70 percent organic.

COSMOS—INTERNATIONAL: "Organic" label: at least 95 percent agro-ingredients; at least 20 percent total product.

COSMEBIO—FRANCE: "Bio" label: at least 95 percent plant-based; at least 10 percent organic.

ECOCERT—INTERNATIONAL: Complies with COSMOS.

ICEA—ITALY: Complies with COSMOS.

IOS: Natural & Organic Cosmetic Standard.

NATURAL PRODUCTS ASSOCIATION (NPA): "Natural" label: at least 95 percent natural.

NSF—US: "Organic" label: at least 70 percent organic.

NATRUE—INTERNATIONAL: "Organic" label: 95 percent organic and 100 percent;

"NATURAL" WITH ORGANIC LABEL: 70 percent organic and 100 percent natural.

OASIS: "Organic": at least 95 percent; "Made with Organic": at least 70 percent.

QUALITY ASSURANCE INTERNATIONAL (QAI)—US: "Made with Organic"; at least 70 percent organic.

SOIL ASSOCIATION—UK: "Organic": at least 95 percent; "Made with Organic": at least 70 percent.

USDA ORGANIC—US: "Organic": at least 95 percent; "Made with Organic": at least 70 percent.

WHOLE FOODS PREMIUM BODY CARE SYMBOL: Products that receive the Premium Body Care Symbol go through rigorous testing in four areas: results, source, environmental impact, and safety (go to *http://www.wholefoodsmarket.com* to access their list of four hundred unacceptable products for body care).

NATURALLY DERIVED AND SYNTHETIC

What does "naturally derived" mean? Like the term "natural," it means different things to different people. "Naturally derived" gives the consumers the impression they are getting a natural product. However, that is often not the case. It may be closer to a synthetic product. What's more, "naturally derived" means that an ingredient started as a whole plant. The problem is that you don't know how many processes it has gone through since it was a whole plant. Often, naturally derived ingredients do not even remotely resemble the original plant they were derived from.

For example, consider cocoamide DEA. This chemical is made using fatty oils from a coconut and processing it with the chemical diethanolamine. A coconut is still considered natural whether it is whole, dried, shredded, or pureed. Oil from the coconut would still be classified as naturally occurring. Once the oil is processed or biochemically altered, it then becomes naturally derived or synthetic, much like cocoamide DEA. If a substance is separated from the whole ingredient and concentrated in a lab, it is considered naturally derived.

Let's look at the terms "natural," "naturally derived," and "synthetic" more closely. A natural chemical is a substance that is derived from mineral, plant, or animal matter and is not processed with synthetics. A synthetic chemical is man-made using methods different from those used in nature. It is the result of two natural chemicals reacting together and making a separate synthetic chemical. By this definition, a synthetic chemical can be made from a natural product and thus be considered as naturally derived. It's highly misleading for even the savviest shopper.

When a company uses the term "naturally derived," it's difficult to know if the ingredient or product is closer to natural or synthetic. Some of these ingredients are truly minimally processed and could be or are classified as natural while others have been processed many times and should not be considered as naturally derived. An ingredient that has been processed once or twice, depending on the processes, can still closely resemble the original natural ingredient. However, ingredients more processed will likely not resemble the original natural source. One may consider an ingredient natural or synthetic depending on the process and how many processes are used. This is what makes this term so confusing. People define this term differently. For the purists, oils and extracts that are distilled, cold-pressed, or otherwise physically separated from plant sources are the only acceptable naturals.

NATURE DERIVED AND NATURE IDENTICAL

"Nature derived" refers to naturally occurring ingredients that are chemically modified to improve their properties in cosmetics. "Nature identical" preservatives are identical to those found in nature but are synthesized in a laboratory. Each of their categories can be considered natural. The health and environmental implications are different.

"Lab identical," also known as "nature identical," is a common ingredient in natural products. Most natural formulas use nature or lab identical preservatives. Totally natural preservatives are difficult to formulate. They require a very specific knowledge to preserve a product. New companies would not be able to enter the natural market if they could not use lab identical preservatives. There are only a few nature-identical preservatives that are permitted in naturals.

Minerals such as mica, iron oxides, and zinc oxide are also lab identical ingredients that are allowed in naturals. The reason is that minerals that are mined are contaminated with other substances. They are rarely found as pure minerals. They must be purified and reestablished in the lab before being formulated into a natural product. Most natural and organic certifiers allow these ingredients in formulas when natural substances cannot be recovered from nature using reasonable technical effort. Nature identical ingredients are 100 percent identical in composition to their counterparts in nature but have been created in the laboratory to ensure stability, safety, and sustainability.

Simply because a product is natural does not mean it is chemically safe. Many people are allergic to natural ingredients. Essential oils have been known to cause rashes and other allergic reactions in some people when applied topically or inhaled. In many cases natural ingredients can be more active than synthetic ingredients. The EWG warns against glycolic acid—which falls under the category of alpha hydroxy acids (AHAs)—a substance naturally derived from sugarcane for its mildly corrosive effects. AHAs are a concern because they are slightly caustic, increase sun sensitivity, and have been associated with long-term cellular damage, and studies have linked them to a potential increased risk of skin cancer. Individuals with nut allergies may have a problem with shea butter or almond oil.

Conversely, not all synthetic chemicals are toxic. Consider this statement from Nneka Leiba, deputy director of research with the EWG, who has been working on EWG's Skin Deep Cosmetics Database for nearly ten years: "Not all [chemicals are bad], but you have to know your stuff and really do your research." This is why I specialize in chemically safe and eco-friendly cosmetics rather than natural or organic. There are some excellent products on the market that are not all natural but are harmless to humans and the environment.

As with all substances natural or synthetic, it is highly individual as to what you can tolerate in your ingredients and in your cosmetic diet. "Chemically safe" is what we are striving for. Still, I believe that in most cases, natural or naturally derived (minimally processed) is best for the individual and the environment.

VEGAN AND GLUTEN-FREE

V egan cosmetics have become increasingly popular, and the movement continues to thrive as many organic cosmetic companies provide vegan cosmetics to increase their customer base. Vegans are strict about what they put into their bodies and what they put on their bodies, including cosmetics and clothes. Again, like the terms "natural" and "organic," the term "vegan" is not regulated. It usually refers to products that do not contain any animal products and that are cruelty free. However, cruelty-free cosmetics are not the same as vegan. Cruelty-free means that the products are not tested on animals, but it does not mean that they are free from animal products. In addition, not all vegan products are organic or natural, so one cannot assume. You need to look for both specifications on the label or packaging.

Here are some nonvegan ingredients to watch out for:

Allantoin	Lanolin
Beeswax	Lard
Carmine	Propolis
Pearl powder	Propylparaben
Collagen	Recaldent *(casein phosphopeptide)*
Elastin	Silk derivatives
Hyaluronic acid	Squalane
Lactose/lactalbumin	Tallow

Gluten is found in grains such as wheat, barley, rye, and oatmeal. Wheat-based ingredients are very common in cosmetics. They are also very difficult to detect. The ingredients are derived from grains but have chemical names, making them hard to spot for the average consumer. For people with gluten sensitivities, this is a problem, as it often causes allergic types of reactions. For those with celiac discase, gluten-free cosmetics are a must. As a result, these people seek out gluten-free cosmetics. Luckily, many cosmetic companies are responding to the demand and are eliminating gluten from their products. Some are labeling, others are providing lists of gluten-free products, and many are excluding it from all their products. (I have provided a list of gluten-free cosmetic companies in Chapter 6.)

One important thing to look for in addition to wheat ingredients is vitamin E. It may be derived from a wheat source and is therefore not gluten-free. Check the label for wheat germ oil.

Here are other gluten ingredients to watch out for:

Barley *(Hordeum distichon)*	Oat *(Avena sativa)*
Corn *(Zea mays)*	Rye
Cyclodextrin	Tocopherol acetate *(vitamin E)*
Dextrin	Triticum vulgare *(wheat)*
Dextrin palmitate	Wheat
Hydrolyzed vegetable protein	Yeast extract
Malt	

CRUELTY-FREE

I am a huge animal lover. I don't believe animals should suffer for beauty. Compassion is beautiful; that's why it is important to me to use cosmetics that do not test on animals. Unfortunately, this term is often used to deceive the consumer. Once again, the term "cruelty-free" is not defined by law, which means it's open to a variety of interpretations. Not all products labeled "cruelty-free" or "not tested on animals" are always what they seem. They may appear as good choices, but that is not always true. Making it more complicated is that many cosmetic companies do not use the term "cruelty-free" in their marketing yet use nonanimal testing methods for their products for safety.

The term "cruelty-free" can be used to imply:

- Neither the product nor its ingredients have ever been tested on animals. This is highly unlikely, however, as almost all ingredients in use today have been tested on animals somewhere, at some time, by someone, and could be tested again.

- While the ingredients have been tested on animals, the final product has not.

- The manufacturer itself did not conduct animal tests but instead relied on a supplier to test for them or relied on another company's previous animal-tested results.

- The testing was done in a foreign country, where laws protecting animals might be weaker than in the United States.

- Either the ingredients or the product have not been tested on animals within the last five, ten, or twenty years (but perhaps were before and could be again).

- Neither the ingredients nor the products have been tested on animals after a certification date and will not be tested on animals in the future.

I have found that the best way to ensure a product is compassionate to animals and truly cruelty-free is to look for the logos of these two companies:

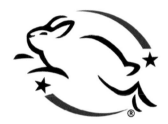

Leaping Bunny: The Coalition for Consumer Information on Cosmetics (CCIC): Established by the Coalition for Consumer Information in Cosmetics (CCIC), a group of eight national animal protection organizations, the Leaping Bunny represents a single, comprehensive standard. Whenever you see this logo, you can be sure that neither the product nor any of its ingredients have been tested on animals. CCIC maintains a Compassionate Shopping Guide of companies that have met their stringent standards. This can be accessed at leapingbunny.org.

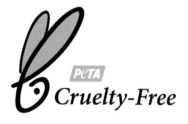

People for Ethical Treatment of Animals (PETA) Beauty without Bunnies: Companies listed have either signed PETA's statement of assurance or provided a statement verifying that they do not conduct, commission, or pay for any tests on animals for ingredients, formulations, or finished products, and that they pledge not to do so in the future. PETA also has a database of companies that do and don't test their products on animals. You can search by company name or browse by product type. There are more than 1,700 cruelty-free companies in their database. You can find this information at peta.org.

Botanical All-Stars

ALGAE/SEAWEED EXTRACT: Rich in beta-carotene, potassium, magnesium, zinc, and iodine.

EVENING PRIMROSE OIL: Loaded with gamma-linolenic acid (GLA) and omega-6 polyunsaturated fatty acids (avoid if you are pregnant or nursing).

GRAPE SEED EXTRACT: Supplies an effective concentration of linoleic acid, which is an omega-6 essential fatty acid, and vitamin E.

GREEN TEA EXTRACT: Packs powerful antioxidants such as catechin and flavonoid polyphenols.

ROSEHIP SEED OIL: Provides potent essentials, such as vitamins A and C, and omega-3 fatty acid.

SEA-BUCKTHORN OIL: Offers a high concentration of omega-7 fatty acid and vitamins A, C, and E.

Chapter Four

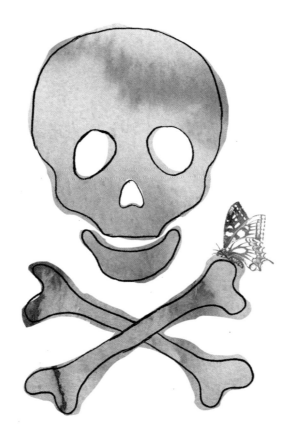

The *Nasties*

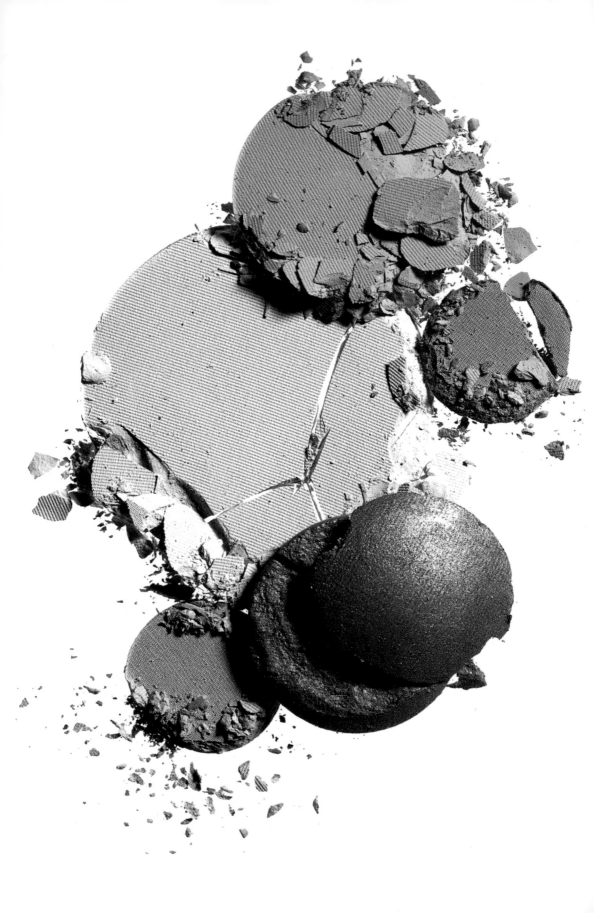

Here comes the heavy—but important—stuff. This is the part many people will want to skip, but please don't. You will want to know about why you should steer clear of petrochemicals, nanoparticles, and certain chemicals that can be toxic depending on how they are used and combined with others. There are many wonderful books about chemicals in cosmetics, and if you want to learn more, I urge you to do so. Here are the highlights and the most important information you need to know.

Most people would be surprised to learn that the 1983 Federal Food, Drug, and Cosmetic Act does not require cosmetics or personal-care products and their ingredients to be approved as safe before they are sold to consumers. The FDA regulates products only after they are sold, investigating health complaints when and if complaints are filed.[3] If you are still asking why you should care about what's in your cosmetics? One word: petrochemicals.

PETROCHEMICALS

The mere word *petrochemical* evokes scary images of tar being slathered onto your skin. Gross! But that's not far from the truth. Petrochemicals are derived from petroleum, natural gas, or coal. The industry started in the 1940s during World War II when there was a demand for synthetic materials to replace costly materials. Since then they have crept into our cosmetics as well. They are found in everything, including shampoos, facial creams, mascaras, perfumes, foundations, and lipsticks—virtually across every cosmetic category.

Petrochemicals appear on labels as mineral oil, petrolatum, and paraffin. They may contain known or suspected human carcinogens and harmful breakdown impurities from the manufacturing process that are not listed on labels, such as dioxin. Petrochemicals found in most cosmetics can be absorbed through the skin and bioaccumulate in the organs and tissues. When this happens, toxic substances continue to accumulate, posing health and environmental risks. Petrochemicals and their byproducts have been known to cause or have been linked to serious health problems, including cancer, neuro and respiratory toxicity, birth defects, and endocrine disruption. They can also cause allergic reactions and skin irritation.

Identify the following petrochemicals by prefixes (the beginning letters) and suffixes (the extensions):

- Chemicals ending in "eth" mean that the petrochemical ethylene oxide was used to produce them. For example, myreth, oleth, laureth, and ceteareth.

- Butanol can be identified with the prefix "butyl." For example, butyl alcohol, butylparaben, and butylene glycol.

- Ethanol can be identified with "ethyl." For example, ethyl alcohol, ethylene glycol, ethylene dichloride, and ethylhexylglycerin, or by the abbreviation EDTA (ethylenediaminetetraacetic acid).

- Methanol can be identified by "methyl" preceding its compound. For example, methyl alcohol, methyl paraben, and methyl cellulose.

- Avoid ingredients containing DEA (diethanolamine) or MEA (monoethanolamine).

- Be alert to ingredients with "propyl." For example, isopropyl alcohol, propylene glycol, propyl alcohol, cocamidopropyl betaine.

CARCINOGENS

arcinogens are substances or exposures that can lead to cancer. Cancer is caused by changes in our DNA at the cellular level. Sometimes the changes occur from the genetics handed down to us from our parents while other changes that occur are caused by outside exposures or environmental factors, such as tobacco use, nutrition, infectious agents, medical treatments, workplace and household exposure, and pollution.[4]

Unfortunately, many of these cancer-causing chemicals are legally allowed in personal care products. The European Union (EU) has banned more than 1,300 toxic chemicals in the EU Cosmetics Directive. The United States has banned only nine. Some carcinogens, such as formaldehyde and 1,4-dioxane, are common in personal care products. Others, while not as common, are still present in our cosmetics and pose a potential health risk.

The International Agency for Research on Cancer (IARC), part of the World Health Organization (WHO), reviews and classifies chemicals into five levels:[5]

Group 1: Carcinogenic to humans	116 agents
Group 2A: Probably carcinogenic to humans	73
Group 2B: Possibly carcinogenic to humans	287
Group 3: Not classifiable as to their carcinogenicity to humans	503
Group 4: Probably not carcinogenic to humans	1

Of the 116 agents listed by IARC as known human carcinogens (Group 1), at least eleven have been or are currently used in personal care products:

- Formaldehyde

- Phenacetin

- Coal tar

- Benzene

- Untreated or mildly treated mineral oils

- Methylene glycol

- Ethylene oxide

- Chromium

- Cadmium (and its compounds)

- Arsenic

- Crystalline silica or quartz[6]

The petrochemical byproduct 1,4-dioxane, recognized as a known human carcinogen in the state of California, is often present in conventional products and those listed as natural and organic. In 2008, a study commissioned by the Organic Consumers Association (OCA), a watchdog group, and overseen by environmental health consumer advocate David Steinman, author of *The Safe Shopper's Bible*, analyzed leading natural and organic brand personal care products for the presence of 1,4-dioxane. Shockingly, the study revealed the toxin was present in leading natural and organic branded products.[7] None of the products with the presence of 1,4-dioxane were certified USDA Organic or BDIH, a nonprofit association of industries and trading firms for pharmaceuticals, health care products, food supplements, and personal hygiene products.

Only one year prior, the EWG found the carcinogen 1,4-dioxane in 28 percent of all personal care products after an exhaustive study of the ingredients in more than 27,000 products.[8] Their investigation found that 1,4-dioxane is a potential contaminant in:

55 percent of baby bubble baths

57 percent of baby shampoos

55 percent of baby soaps

43 percent of body-firming lotions

37 percent of antiaging lotions

35 percent of around-eye creams

ENDOCRINE DISRUPTORS

Endocrine disruptors are also known as estrogenic chemicals or substances. They disrupt the endocrine system, a network of glands and hormones that regulate many bodily functions. These glands produce hormones that are released into the bloodstream, relaying information to different parts of the body. Endocrine disruptors interfere with growth, development, intelligence, and reproduction.

Our bodies are continuously exposed to hundreds of estrogenic chemicals on a daily basis. Some are natural, such as lavender and tea tree oil, while others are not. Natural estrogen is called phytoestrogen. Plants produce chemicals that mimic and interact with the estrogen in our bodies. These estrogens, such as estradiol or synthetic hormones used in birth control pills or hormone replacement therapy, are generally thought to be weaker than the ones we produce naturally.

Our exposure is mainly through our diet, as they are in many of the foods we eat, including herbs, seasonings, grains, fruits, and vegetables. Those that are not phytoestrogens are potential endocrine disruptors that interfere with our body's normal functions. They can keep estrogen levels continually high and above the natural levels. When this happens, problems can surface.

Some common ingredients in cosmetics that are associated with endocrine disruption include parabens, phthalates, BHA and BHT, and resorcinol (for a full list, see section to follow).

Gender Benders

8-PRENYLNARINGENIN

This chemical is found in the female flowers of the hops plant. It has long been used as a preservative and a flavoring agent in beer, but it is now being found in some herbal preparations for women for breast enhancement. It mimics estrogen activity, increasing the production rates of many types of human breast cancer cells.

ALUMINUM SALTS

These are a form of metal and work by blocking the pores that produce perspiration. They are found in antiperspirants and may be listed in the ingredients on the bottle as aluminum chlorohydrate or aluminum zirconium. They can be measured in the blood following application to human underarms. They are endocrine disruptors. Endocrine disruptors are chemicals that interfere with the endocrine (or hormone) system in animals and can cause cancerous tumors, birth defects, and other developmental disorders.

BHA AND BHT

Used mainly in moisturizers and makeup as preservatives. Suspected endocrine disruptors and may cause cancer (BHA). Encourages the breakdown of vitamins such as vitamin D; can cause lipid and cholesterol levels to increase, is an endocrine disruptor, and is toxic.

COAL TAR

This is a black, viscid liquid distilled from coal and used to make a variety of products, from dyes to pavements. It can cause cancer and may interfere with reproductive development. It can be found in shampoos, dandruff scalp treatments, and anti-itch rash creams.

CYCLOSILOXANES

These are the building blocks for many silicones. Some widely used ones are: hexamethylcyclotrisiloxane (D3), octamethylcyclotetrasiloxane (D4), decamethylcyclopentasiloxane (D5), and dodecamethylcyclohexasiloxane (D6). They mimic estrogen activity, increasing the production rates of many types of human breast cancer cells. They can be found in hair conditioners.

DIBUTYL PHTHALATE (DBP)

These plasticizers, substances added to plastics to increase their flexibility, transparency, durability, and longevity, have been linked to breast cancer and reproductive developmental problems. They can be found in products including nail polish, moisturizer, eye shadow, and fragrances.

FORMALDEHYDE

This preservative may cause cancer and interfere with reproductive development. It may be found in moisturizers, facial cleansers, shampoos, conditioners, body washes, eye shadows, mascaras, nail treatments, and flame-retardant products. It's harmful to the immune system and is a known human carcinogen.

HYDROQUINONE

This aromatic organic compound is an active ingredient in several skin creams that are used for depigmentation of melasma—pigmented areas—age spots and scars. It can be cancer causing and may interfere with reproductive development. It is often found in skin fader/lighteners, hair bleach and colors, facial moisturizer/treatments, and powders.

MIROESTROL/DEOXYMIROESTROL

These phytoestrogens, or plant-derived chemicals that mimic the biological activity of the hormone estrogen, can be found in breast enhancers. They mimic estrogen activity, increasing the production rates of many types of human breast cancer cells.

PARABENS

These synthetic preservatives have been linked to breast and prostate cancer. They are considered an illegal ingredient in Europe. They can be found in cosmetics such as shampoos, conditioners, body washes, tooth whiteners, toothpastes, facial cleansers, sunscreens, moisturizers, and astringents.

PLACENTAL EXTRACT

Highly estrogenic as it is taken from the placenta of a female mammal, this is used in some skin and hair products. The Skin Deep Cosmetics Database cites that in one study, four girls between one and eight years of age developed breasts or pubic hair two to twenty-four months after starting the use of estrogen- or placenta-containing hair products. Their breasts and pubic hair regressed when they stopped using the products.

SUNSCREENS (BENZOPHENONES)

These absorb ultraviolet light. However, they also penetrate the human skin and mimic estrogen activity, increasing the production rates of many types of human breast cancer cells. They can be found in sunscreens and cosmetics with sunscreen in them under the ingredients labeled 3-(4-methylbenzylidene)-camphor (4-MBC), octyl-methoxycinnamate (OMC), octyl-dimethyl-PABA (OD-PABA), benzophenone-3 (Bp-3), and homosalate (HMS).

TOLUENE

This is a clear, water-insoluble liquid with the typical smell of paint thinners. It is a common solvent, able to dissolve paints, paint thinners, silicone sealants, many chemical reactants, rubber, printing ink, adhesives (glues), lacquers, leather tanners, and disinfectants. High amounts of toluene can lead to birth defects, developmental abnormalities, and cancer. It may appear on ingredient labels as phenyl-methane, methylbenzene, or toluol and can be found in nail polish and treatments.

TRICLOSAN

This antibacterial agent may block the metabolism of thyroid hormone by chemically mimicking it and binding to the hormone receptor sites, blocking them, so that normal hormones cannot be used. It also contributes to antibiotic resistance. It is found in a variety of products, including moisturizers, hand creams, shampoos, conditioners, liquid soaps, antiperspirants, and toothpastes.

GLYCOL ETHERS

The European Union says that some of these chemicals may damage fertility or the unborn child.

RESORCINOL

Used in hair color, hair care products, and skin care; specifically used to treat acne and antiaging and other dermatological uses. In higher doses it has been shown to disrupt the endocrine system, specifically thyroid function; disrupt the function of the central nervous system; and lead to respiratory problems. This common ingredient is toxic to the immune system. The federal government regulates exposures to resorcinol in the workplace, but there is no regulation restricting the use of resorcinol in personal care products.

Antiaging Decoded

The Old Guard: Chemicals to Avoid or Use with Caution

VITAMIN A DERIVATIVES RETINYL PALMITATE, RETINYL ACETATE, RETINOIC ACID, AND RETINOL are used in daytime products such as sunscreens and hydrators.

ALPHA AND BETA HYDROXY ACIDS (AHAs/BHAs) are glycolic and lactic acid and are used to exfoliate, retexturize, and smooth skin.

HYDROQUINONE is used as a skin-lightening agent. The FDA warns that it can cause a skin disease called ochronosis.

The New Guard: Healthy Antiaging Ingredients

COENZYME Q10 is naturally made in our bodies to neutralize free radicals in cells.

HYALURONIC ACID is a natural compound found in skin that helps retain moisture, plump up skin, and alleviate fine lines and wrinkles.

VITAMIN C helps stimulate the production of collagen and minimize fine lines, wrinkles, and scars.

CERAMIDE is naturally found in the skin cells and helps retain moisture and plumps the skin, giving it a more youthful appearance.

RESVERATROL is a natural compound produced by plants and is packed with antioxidants that combat signs of aging.

PEPTIDES are chains of amino acids that are the building blocks of proteins in the skin. Peptides can prompt the formation of new collagen.

NIACINAMIDE is made from niacin, also known as vitamin B3. It works to improve skin's elasticity, eliminate discoloration, and revive tone and texture.

Vitamin A: Hype or Hero?

Hero (sort of). This little guy should be wearing a mask and cape. Vitamin A in all its forms—retinyl palmitate, retinol, and retinoids—is the antiaging superhero ingredient. It works! Period. Vitamin A dramatically reduces fine lines and wrinkles, gives the skin a smooth texture, and evens out skin tone, imparting an overall youthful appearance. But that's just the highlights. It's also a powerful antioxidant and can help with more than a hundred skin issues.[9] Sounds like the fountain of youth, right?

Retinol is the synthetic form of vitamin A. Retinoids are more potent compounds that are broken down from retinol. Retinoids, such as tretinoin (brand name Retin-A), are available by prescription, whereas retinol can be purchased over the counter. Retinyl palmitate, weaker than retinol, is also available over the counter and often labeled vitamin A.

Here's the bad news. The FDA has classified retinol as a known human reproductive toxicant. Retinol/retinyl esters are also listed on California's Proposition 65 list for developmental toxicity.[10] The EWG Skin Deep Cosmetics Database ranks it a 9, a high hazard. Furthermore, vitamin A is extremely toxic in high doses. The bummer for me is that any vitamin A or derivative ingredient will drive up a score on a perfectly low, clean, and safe product on the database. Many amazing antiaging products will rank higher than 3 because they contain vitamin A.

This poses a huge dilemma. Should we or shouldn't we? Here's how I feel about the situation. If you really feel you must use it, use it with caution. Never use day wear products with retinol or vitamin A–derived ingredients. Also, be mindful of how often and when you are using it. Vitamin A and its derivatives make you photosensitive and increase your chances of getting sunburned. Combined with other products such as glycolic and lactic acid, it will increase skin sensitivity and could irritate your skin. Absorption enhancers will drive the ingredient deeper into your skin. Factor it in your daily 80/20 chemical intake.

As I write this book, I am not using any retinol or retinoids. However, I have thought about it recently and decided against it. Here's why. I am happy with the way my skin looks right now. I prefer the way my skin looks without it. Right now my skin looks fleshy and plump. I used Retin-A when I was a teenager and in my twenties. I loved it. I had acne, and it really controlled it. In high school I was on Accutane (three times). Yikes. That was rough too. I hated the side effects but loved not having acne. I had much more confidence with clear skin, and there's something to be said for that. If I had acne, I would use Retin-A again. For me, the benefits outweighed the risks, but as it stands now, for antiaging it doesn't.

Toxic Chemicals to Avoid for Women with Medium to Dark Skin Tones

- **BHA** (relaxers, skin lighteners, hair-growth products)
- **COAL TAR** (hair dyes)
- **COUMARIN** (hair dyes, hair relaxers)
- **DMDM HYDANTOIN** (hair relaxers, hair dyes, skin lighteners)
- **FORMALDEHYDE** (hair straighteners, nail care)
- **HYDROQUINONE** (skin care, hair dyes)
- **PLACENTAL EXTRACT** (skin care, hair care)

NANOPARTICLES AND TITANIUM DIOXIDE

Nanoparticles are particles that are so small, they are measured in nanometers. For those of us who aren't math geniuses, that is billionths of a meter. These megafine particles have been wonderfully helpful for the cosmetic industry. The tiny little bits actually "fill in" the skin's crevices and result in an ultrasmooth finish. Formulas that include nanoparticles are lustrous and provide a sumptuous look and feel to the product and skin. While it does produce a highly desired, fine quality, and it is gorgeous, it can also present a serious health risk when inhaled or absorbed through the skin. When nanoparticles are inhaled, they can get trapped in the respiratory system and deposit on the lungs. This can be a health risk for anyone, especially those with bronchial-related health issues. Loose powders and mineral makeup often include nanoparticles. Some manufacturers list the nanoparticle ingredient while others do not.

Titanium dioxide is used extensively in loose and pressed cosmetic powders as a whitening agent. Powdered and ultrafine titanium dioxide dust is a carcinogen that has been implicated in respiratory tract cancer in rats exposed during laboratory testing. In 2006 the International Agency for Research on Cancer classified titanium dioxide as a carcinogen.[11]

Micronized ingredients are not necessarily nanoparticles. Micronized ingredients are measured in millionths of a meter, not billionths like nanoparticles, which makes a micron one thousand times larger than a nanometer. Unfortunately, there is no way to know what you are getting unless the label states "micronized" or "nanoparticle."

Like so much of the information available in the cosmetic industry, it is difficult to know which cosmetic products do not have nanoparticles if they are not listed. This is one reason the EWG warns against loose powders and titanium dioxide in any formulas that can be inhaled, such as loose powders or sprays.

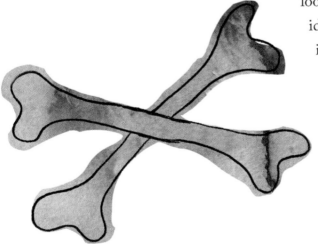

READING LABELS: BE A "BOX TURNER"

Here are some simple rules for reading ingredient labels:

RULE 1: Read from top to bottom (↓). Companies generally list ingredients in order of quantity (greatest to least). The ingredients listed first will constitute the highest percentage in the product. If the first ingredients are petrochemicals and the natural ingredients are at the bottom of the list, you'll probably want to leave the product on the shelf. Ingredients with concentrations lower than 1 percent may be listed in any order. Labels do not indicate where high-concentration ingredients end and where low-concentration ingredients begin.

RULE 2: The more ingredients listed, the more concerned you should be. This is not always the case, but often it is. When I see that only three natural ingredients were used to make the product, I know it is clean.

RULE 3: Exercise caution with long names that are difficult to pronounce. Safe cosmetics will list common names next to their scientific name. For example, aloe vera's scientific name is *Aloe barbadensis*. Products with natural ingredients list both names.

RULE 4: Know that products may list "trade secret" as an ingredient. This can be deceptive. A trade secret is a legal nondisclosure term allowing the manufacturer to protect any formula that gives the product a competitive advantage. Examples are lipstick colors and fragrance. Fragrance may contain hundreds of toxic chemicals that do not have to be disclosed, since under trade secret, the formula is proprietary.

Naturally derived fragrances do not use fragrance (parfum or perfume), but a specific naming system. If you are trying to avoid certain chemicals, they may be present in trade secret products that are not being disclosed.

RULE 5: Understand that when ingredients share the same name there is no distinction between what is produced naturally or synthetically. The same chemical can be derived synthetically or naturally. The way ingredients are derived is seldom listed on the label.

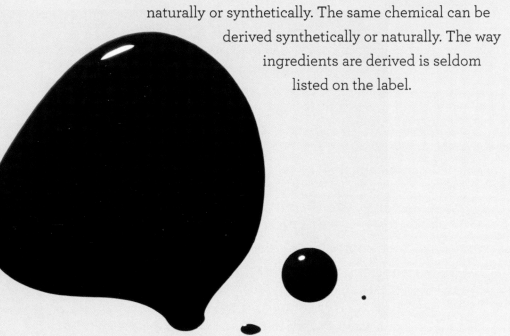

THE NASTIES: TWENTY OF THE MOST COMMON TOXIC CHEMICALS FOUND IN COSMETICS

1. **1,4-DIOXANE,** a byproduct of the manufacturing process when the chemical petrochemical ethylene oxide is introduced, is considered a probable human carcinogen by the US Environmental Protection Agency (EPA). The best you can do is to look for chemicals with "eth" in their name, such as sodium laureth sulfate, oleth, myreth, and ceteareth. Also look for glycol and PEGs (polyethylene, polyethylene glycol, and polyoxyethylene).

2. **SODIUM LAURYL SULFATE (SLS) AND SODIUM LAURYL ETHER SULFATE (SLES)** are coconut-derived foaming agents. These chemicals are used in a wide variety of hair care and skin care products. SLS is a proven skin irritant and possible carcinogen. It alters skin structure, allowing other chemicals deeper penetration and therefore increasing the amount of chemicals in the bloodstream. SLES contains the carcinogen contaminant 1,4-dioxane.

3. **FRAGRANCE (PARFUM OR PERFUME)** is a ubiquitous term often used to mask the use of hundreds of toxic chemicals. It's used in cosmetics and household products. Upward of three hundred chemicals in this class have never been tested for safety, including phthalates, which disrupt endocrine function and have been linked to reproductive and developmental harm.

4. **PARABENS (METHYL, ETHYL, PROPYL, AND BUTYL)** are used in about 99 percent of beauty products to prevent oxidation, kill bacteria, and other living organisms harmful to humans. They are rapidly absorbed into the skin and metabolize and

accumulate in the body. Parabens disrupt endocrine function by mimicking estrogen. Improper endocrine function can adversely affect metabolism, the nervous system, and blood sugar levels.

5. **TRICLOSAN** is used in almost all antibacterial products. It's used as a preservative in soaps, toothpaste, and cosmetics. Triclosan is often contaminated with dioxins that are carcinogenic, weaken immunity, decrease fertility, and cause birth defects. A probable endocrine disruptor, triclosan is easily absorbed, leading to bioaccumulation at dangerous levels.

6. **HYDROQUINONE** is commonly found in skin lighteners and facial moisturizers. It is an allergen, immune system and respiratory toxicant, probable neurotoxin, and possible carcinogen. Animal studies show endocrine disruption.

7. **TALC** is used in many cosmetics, such as powdered eye shadow and blush, and is a carcinogenic link between talcum powder and ovarian cancer. Talc contaminated with asbestos can cause lung tumors and is a probable respiratory toxin.

8. **PHTHALATES** are a class of toxic chemicals used in cosmetics to hold color and scent, and to soften plastics. They are found in products ranging from fragranced lotions, body wash, and deodorants to most plastic containers. These chemicals are known reproductive toxicants. Phthalates mimic estrogen and testosterone, increasing the risk for endocrine disruption.

9. **FORMALDEHYDE/FORMALIN** is an immune system, respiratory, hematological, and skin toxicant. It is a probable carcinogen, cardiovascular toxicant, can damage DNA, and may trigger asthma. Animal studies show adverse effects on sense organs, the brain and nervous system, and human development.

10. **COAL TAR** is used in dandruff shampoos and anti-itch creams. Coal tar–based dyes, such as FD&C Blue 1, are used in toothpaste, while FD&C Green 3 is used in mouthwash. This chemical is a known carcinogen, and a skin and respiratory toxicant.

11. **DMDM HYDANTOIN** is an antimicrobial formaldehyde releaser that is useful as a preservative. It is used in hair products, cosmetics, skin oils and moisturizers, sunscreen, and even baby wipes. DMDM hydantoin is a known human allergen and immune toxicant, causing irritation to the skin, eyes, and lungs, and is a possible carcinogen.

12. **TRIETHANOLAMINE (TEA)** is used primarily as an emulsifier and surfactant, both useful for binding water with oil. This chemical is commonly used in products such as mascara, styling gel, hand cream, and laundry detergent. It is both an immune system and respiratory system toxicant, and skin allergen.

13. **POLYETHYLENE GLYCOL (PEG)** is a petroleum derivative compound that is made from ethylene glycol (ethane-1,2-diol), the main ingredient found in antifreeze. It is used to prevent foaming, and in cosmetics as a thickener and softener. PEGs can be contaminated with ethylene oxide and 1,4-dioxane, which is harmful to the nervous system and a possible carcinogen.

14. **ALPHA AND BETA HYDROXY ACIDS (AHAS AND BHAS)** are used in cosmetics as antiaging agents. The concern is that application of acids to the skin destroys the upper layers of skin. This process irritates the skin, leading to burns, permanent scarring, permanent UV damage, and probable increased risk for cancer.

15. **SYNTHETIC DYES** appear on the ingredients label as FD&C or D&C, and are used to provide color for products such as shampoo, makeup, pharmaceuticals, and food. Synthetic dyes are probable carcinogens. When present, these chemicals will appear as FD&C or D&C followed by a color and a number like Red No. 6 or Green No. 6.

16. **ALUMINUM ZIRCONIUM** and other aluminums are compounds often used in eye shadow as a color additive and most commonly found in antiperspirant deodorants. This ingredient blocks pores, which prevents sweat from leaving the body. Aluminum in ionic forms is carcinogenic, toxic, and mutagenic. Aluminum salts mimic estrogen and have been linked to breast cancer.

17. **OXYBENZONE** is a chemical used in sunscreen for the purpose of UV protection. It is a bioaccumulate, possible immune toxicant, endocrine disruptor, and allergen. Oxybenzone is also used in antiaging cream, conditioner, lip balm, and lipstick.

18. **LAURAMIDE DEA (SAME AS COCAMIDE MEA)** is a coconut oil–derived diethanolamine used as a foaming agent and emulsifying agent. Lauramide DEA or cocamide MEA is a human immune toxicant. Animal studies show that this chemical is linked to sense organ effects and skin irritation.

19. **DIETHANOLAMINE (DEA)** is a chemical used as a wetting agent in shampoos, lotions, creams, and other cosmetics. It is a skin and immune toxicant, and possible carcinogen. Animal studies show DEA linked to endocrine disruption and neurotoxicity.

20. **TOLUENE** is useful for suspending color in nail polish, nail treatments, hair color, and hair bleach. In nail products, toluene forms a smooth finish across the nails. Toluene is a respiratory toxicant, skin irritant, and probable human development toxicant.

NAVIGATE THE NASTIES USING YOUR ECO-ATTITUDE

That's a pretty big list, right? I know it's daunting to read labels and understand what everything means. I don't want you to feel overwhelmed thinking you need to remember every chemical. For me, the easiest way to remember things is to keep it simple. In Chapter 1 you chose your eco-attitude. You were either a Green Beauty Beginner, Pro, or Master. You didn't think that was all just for fun, did you? It's actually a really useful tool. Your eco-attitude will determine what products to eliminate at your individual stage.

1. **GREEN BEAUTY BEGINNER:** You are ready to jump on the Filthy Five bandwagon. I selected the first five chemicals for you because these are among the first to be taken out of many so-called green products, as well as traditional ones. These chemicals are also easy to identify, so you won't have to overthink when you are trying to determine whether these toxins have been excluded—you can immediately go back to looking pretty.

2. **GREEN BEAUTY PRO:** You begin your transition to clean at the Dirty Dozen level. I chose the first twelve chemicals based on an interview I did with Nneka Leiba, deputy director of research with the EWG. Leiba cited parabens and fragrance in her list for the top chemicals of most concern in personal care products.

3. **GREEN BEAUTY MASTER:** Your journey starts with the Toxic Twenty. This list contains some of the most common toxic cosmetic chemicals. The spirit of the Green Beauty Master is more of a purist. You'll want to eliminate toxic chemicals and replace them with quality ingredients such as nut oil, fruit extracts, antioxidants, and vitamins. You'll be happiest with fewer ingredients and names that you can easily pronounce and identify.

Remember, there is no one list that will give you all the toxic chemicals you should avoid, but these are some of the most common ones. The website Teens Turning Green (*http://www.teensturninggreen .org/*) has a Dirty Thirty list of toxic chemicals to avoid.

Green Beauty Beginner **The Filthy Five**	1. Fragrance (parfum/perfume) 2. Parabens (methyl, ethyl, propyl, and butyl) 3. Talc (especially in loose powder) 4. Sodium lauryl sulfate (SLS) Sodium lauryl ether sulfate (SLES) 5. Triclosan
Green Beauty Pro **The Dirty Dozen**	6. Hydroquinone 7. 1,4-dioxane 8. Phthalates 9. Formaldehyde/formalin 10. Coal tar 11. DMDM hydantoin 12. Triethanolamine (TEA)
Green Beauty Master **The Toxic Twenty**	13. Polyethylene glycol (PEG) 14. Alpha and beta hydroxy acids (AHAs and BHAs) 15. Synthetic dyes 16. Aluminum zirconium and other aluminum compounds 17. Oxybenzone 18. Lauramide DEA (same as cocamide MEA) 19. Diethanolamine (DEA) 20. Toluene

THE THREE Ps

No matter what your eco-attitude, when in doubt, remember the Three Ps and avoid these chemicals as often as you can:

1. **PARABENS:** Look for the prefixes methyl, propyl, ethyl, butyl, and isopropyl.

2. **PERFUME:** Look for parfum or fragrance.

3. **PETROCHEMICALS:** Look for the abbreviations PEG, DEA, and SLS, as well as any ingredients with an *x* or *y*, for example, ethylhexylglycerin.

I know we covered a lot in this chapter, but don't feel overwhelmed. As I said, you don't need to memorize all the chemicals. For now, just get familiar with them, especially those in your overall eco-attitude. Look at the chemicals in the other eco-attitudes as well, since you will no doubt bounce between them. Use them as a guide and refer to them when you need to. Many of them will soon become part of your daily vocabulary while others may stick with you after some time as you shop and seek out chemically safe products. I use these eco-attitudes nearly every time I shop. I ask myself: *What do I need it for? How important is performance? How much am I willing to spend? When do I need it? How much time do I have to shop and is convenience important?* How I answer these questions will dictate which eco-attitude I have adopted. I have found that I live as a Green Beauty Pro but dip into the Green Beauty Master attitude quite often and the Green Beauty Beginner attitude occasionally.

SKIP THE DIP: Say "no" when you are offered
a paraffin dip at a spa or nail salon. Paraffin wax is
another word for petrochemical.

These Substances Are Toxic
When Inhaled

- **TALC** (makeup)

- **TITANIUM DIOXIDE** (makeup)

- **SILICONE-DERIVED CHEMICALS** (skin care, hair care, makeup)

- **MICA** (makeup)

- **NANOPARTICLES** (sunscreen, skin care)

- **MANGANESE VIOLET** (makeup)

The Green Teen:
Toxic Chemicals for Teens to Avoid

1. **PARABENS:** hormone disruptor, found in 99 percent of
   cosmetics.

2. **FRAGRANCE:** hormone disruptor, found in a vast majority
   of cosmetics, including skin care, body care, makeup, and
   hair care.

3. **TRICLOSAN:** hormone disruptor, found in body care, skin care,
   and oral care.

4. **TOLUENE:** hormone disruptor, found in nail polish.

5. **OXYBENZONE:** hormone disruptor, found in sunscreen, skin
   care, and lip balms.

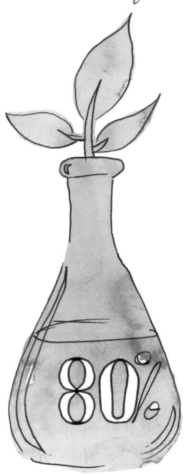

Chapter Five

TRANSITION to
Clean:
Forty-Eight Hours
to Toxic-Free Cosmetics

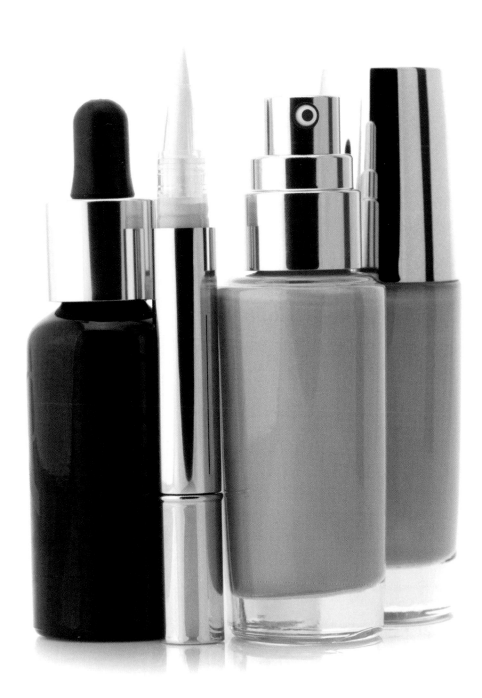

This is the part of the book where you "do" rather than simply read. It's where all the action takes place. Get ready to dig in. You are two days away from a green beauty routine. How great is that? Yesterday, it was only a wish. Today, with my guidance, it's about to happen for real! Not only that, you'll be well prepared to do it on your own. You'll be equipped with all the information and tools you need to confidently integrate your favorite products, read labels with savvy, identify toxic chemicals, and shop like a pro! You will no longer wonder if a product is really natural or a company is the real deal—you'll know!

DAY 1:
Take Stock—Your EWG Scores

CONSIDER DAY 1 LIKE SPRING-CLEANING for your cosmetics and personal care products. It is all about taking stock, analyzing, and purging. You are going to scrutinize and evaluate your own personal care products by getting savvy with EWG's Skin Deep Cosmetics Database and surveying your favorite ten products to see which ones can be saved and which ones are deal breakers and have to go. If your favorite products don't make the cut, I will provide options for replacing them in Chapter 7. Be prepared to potentially give up at least a couple of products immediately.

Now pull out that magnifying glass, because you're going to be reading lots of labels. Make sure you've blocked out a few hours to devote to this, but remember that you only have to do this once. If you take the time to do this right, you'll never again need to dedicate this much time to having clean products.

STEP 1 **Collect all your cosmetics, including anything you use for beautification or hygiene.** Gather everything from your bathroom cabinets, cosmetic bags and travel cases, shower and bath, and storage cabinets in your hallways. Make sure to include all items from across all categories (makeup, skin care, body, hair, oral, sun care, personal/feminine care, etc.).

STEP 2 **Immediately toss products you don't need to keep.** Toss anything that:

1. Is old or broken.
2. Has expired (see the sidebar When to Toss Out Makeup).
3. Hasn't been used in six months.
4. Is empty.

When to Toss Out Makeup

The best way to tell if a product has gone bad is by using your senses. You will know better than any expiration date. The way it smells, looks, and tastes will give you enough information about its stability. If doesn't smell right, starts to separate, develops little beads, or tastes funky, it's gone off. Time to toss it! As a general rule, the more moisture and the closer it gets to your eyes, the shorter the shelf life it will have. You can't always tell when bacteria is building up. It's a good idea to replace your products regularly. Get your trash can ready and refer to this guide:

Makeup Shelf Life

- **Foundation:** one year
- **Concealer:** one year
- **Powders:** two years
- **Lipstick:** one year
- **Lip gloss:** one year
- **Lip liner:** one year
- **Liquid eyeliner:** three months
- **Eyeliner gel:** six months
- **Eyeliner pencil:** one year
- **Mascara:** three months

STEP 3 **Think about your grooming rituals and prioritize the top ten products you use most on a daily basis.** For example, shampoos, conditioners, soaps, body washes, makeup, skin care, and body hydrators are common daily use products. Which products do you use on a daily basis? Separate these products from the others. For example, following is a list of products I use on a daily basis.

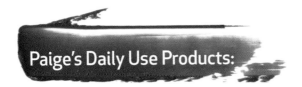

Paige's Daily Use Products:

1. Toothpaste
2. Facial hydrator
3. Body wash/soap
4. Lip balm
5. Deodorant
6. Nail polish
7. Concealer
8. Mascara
9. Bronzer/contour
10. Facial Cleanser
11. Eye cream
12. Serum/treatment

Your selection will be different than mine, but you'll share common products with my list. Also, think about the cosmetics you love the most—the ones you can't live without. Is there anything you can't give up, like a signature scent, for instance? That perfect mascara that lengthens and volumizes? A luxurious eye cream that lifts and firms? However you answer, these will most likely be your cheat products, or what I like to call your ice-cream sundae. These cosmetics are your 20 percent toxic chemical allowance. Put these products aside and we'll deal with them later.

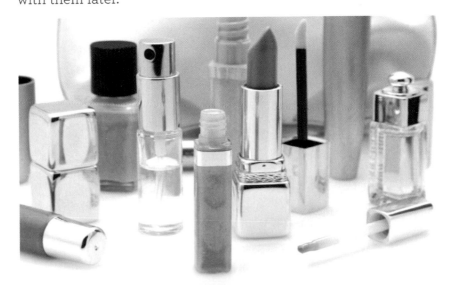

STEP 4   **Looking at your stash of products you use on a daily basis, now you are going to determine which products to replace first, and the point at which you need to replace the remaining ones.** I recommend you replace these daily use products first based on warnings from the EWG:

Perfume/fragrance, including body mists and synthetic oils. Fragrance may contain hundreds of toxic chemicals. Phthalates, which are linked to birth defects in boys, are commonly found in fragrance.

Skin lighteners, especially those containing hydroquinone, are some of the most toxic products you will use. Hydroquinone is a known carcinogen and is banned in Canada and the European Union.

Loose powder, especially those with talc and titanium dioxide. Talc has been linked to acute and chronic lung irritation. Titanium dioxide is a possible carcinogen when inhaled. Loose powders, especially face powders and mineral makeup, commonly use titanium dioxide in their formulas.

DIY: Fix Any Broken Powder

Has your pristine new blush or bronzer ever shattered to bits? Your favorite eye shadow started to crack and crumble? It's such a bummer to throw away a powder you love simply because it's been broken—not to mention it can be expensive to replace. The good news is you don't have to throw away broken eye shadow or pressed powder. You can fix it in minutes with only one ingredient: rubbing alcohol. Don't worry; it's a low toxic hazard.

1. Crush all the broken powder into its original component.

2. Once you've crumbled the powder, add a few drops of rubbing alcohol.

3. Smooth the powder and alcohol with your finger. If you prefer, you can cover the component with plastic wrap first to protect your finger. Once it's smooth, remove the wrap.

4. If you are repairing an eye shadow, place a quarter on top of the powder and press firmly to pack the powder and create a smooth surface. Remove the coin. If you are repairing a larger compact you can use the bottom of a drinking glass.

5. Let the powder dry. It may dry in a few hours, but letting it dry overnight is best. You can use water instead of alcohol, but it will take much longer to dry.

Should You Replace a Product?

If you're undecided on whether or not to replace a product, use these four qualifying questions to help you:

1. What do I need it for?

2. How clean am I right now in my beauty routine?

3. How many ingredients are unknown or potentially toxic and where do they fall on the ingredient list?

4. Does it include any of the Three Ps?

I know you may not be thrilled at the thought of giving up one or several of these products. I wasn't either—at first. I had dreadful images of myself with an oily T-zone, sunspots all over my face and chest, and never smelling irresistible again. Then, after the feelings of panic subsided, I made a decision. Rather than feel as though I could never use any of these beauty items ever again, I would consider these warnings in my decision to use them if I felt I must.

Here is what I did: I gave up loose face powder (for the most part). Occasionally, I use loose powder brighteners and loose powders that do not contain titanium dioxide or talc. I admit this wasn't hard for me to give up, as I prefer to work with pressed powders in general. I no longer use any lightening products with hydroquinone. Instead, I look for ingredients such as licorice, kojic acid, and niacinamide. These can be just as effective, especially when combined. Keep reading, and I will tell you how I allow myself to use fragrance and how you can keep your favorite lipstick!

STEP 5   **Check and record the scores of your products using the EWG's Skin Deep Cosmetics Database.** I want you to look up all the products you use on a daily basis. But before you do this, get the app (see the sidebar Six Free Apps)! If you download the EWG's app onto your smartphone, you'll find that it has a handy time-saving scanner, and you will wonder how you ever lived without it. If you don't have a smartphone, don't stress. You can still do this. The scanner is a bonus and makes the process quicker, but it's not essential. You can also log on to their website (*http://www.ewg.org/skindeep*) and input ingredient names directly into their online database using the Build Your Own Report tool.

Six Free Apps You Should Have on Your Smart Phone

1. EWG's SKIN DEEP COSMETICS DATABASE: A nice addition to the EWG Skin Deep Cosmetic Database. This scanner can save you time while shopping (*www.ewg.org/skindeep*).

2. TOTAL BEAUTY: Read reviews of hundreds of products, many of which are natural. I love the built-in shopping feature (*www.totalbeauty.com*)!

3. LEAPING BUNNY: Find cosmetic companies that are cruelty-free. What's best, you can search by company or category (*leapingbunny.org*).

4. AUBREY "DICTIONARY OF COMMON TERMS": A handy cosmetic ingredients dictionary and key ingredients section keep me engrossed for hours (*www.aubrey-organics.com*).

5. EWG's SUNSCREEN GUIDE: Find the best safe sunscreens or look up your sunscreen. The sun safety tips are a nice bonus (*www.ewg.org/sunscreen*).

6. THE GOODGUIDE: This app allows you to search product categories and offers you alternative for products containing ingredients you want to eliminate (*www.goodguide.com*).

EWG is a nonprofit, nonpartisan organization that publishes valuable information to protect human health and the environment. It is the authority on toxic chemicals in the environment and in cosmetics. The database currently has more than 70,000 products, but it fluctuates between 60,000 and 70,000, with new products being added and old ones deleted. It's easy to navigate, and you can look up a product, ingredients, product lines, or companies. You can also find replacements for your traditional makeup by searching categories such as "foundation" or "body lotion."

I have been referring to their website for ten years and using their database since 2006. EWG's ratings represent the best available data on the safety of personal care product ingredients. It has shaped my green beauty philosophy and helped me green my personal and professional kits. While I can't follow all their warnings all the time, I do consider them with every purchase I make. The highest scoring products are the most toxic, so replace them first. Then replace your daily use products according to EWG's hazard score.

For the purposes of this book, this is how the hazard score system works:*

Score of 3 or lower: The product is fine to keep.

Scores of 4–6: Replace the product with a clean alternative as soon as it runs out.

Score 7 or higher: Replace the product immediately!

*The EWG ranks products scoring 2 or less as low and 3–6 as moderate. I am a little more forgiving since it can be difficult to find cosmetics ranking a 2 or lower. But if you have a large number of products that score a 3, you should consider looking for replacements for some of them. Besides, in chapter 7 I give you tons of chemically safe and high performance beauty products that rank a 2 or lower you you'll have all your basics and core products figured out for you.

The following products mentioned are actual products I use. However, I am constantly changing my products to try new ones so that

I may share them with you. Here are my EWG scores based on my daily use products given earlier:

Paige's Beauty Routine Scores from EWG's Skin Deep Cosmetics Database		
1. Toothpaste	Tom's of Maine Antiplaque & Whitening Flouride-Free Natural Toothpaste, Fennel	1
2. Facial hydrator	Luminance Facial Moisturizer Hydration	1*
3. Body wash	Shea Moisture Coconut & Hibiscus Foaming Milk BodyWash	2
4. Lip balm	S.W. Basics	0
5. Deodorant	Thai Crystal Deodorant Stone	1
6. Nail polish	Deborah Lippmann Nail Color, Fashion	2
7. RMS Beauty	'Un' Cover-up	1
8. Mascara	W3ll People Expressionist Bio Extreme Mascara	3
9. Bronzer/contour	ZuZu Luxe Bronzer Matte	2
10. Facial Cleanser	Ecco Bella Cleansing Milk & Makeup Remover	1
11. Eye cream	Weleda Pomegranate Firming Eye Cream	1
12. Serum/treatment	Tammy Fender Quintessential Serum	0*

Not listed in EWG database; scored with Build Your Own Report tool.

As you can see, my daily beauty routine is pretty clean. The mascara ranks a 3, a low-moderate concern on the database. I allow it because I know it's clean overall. The ingredients that drive up the score are fragrance chemicals (geraniol, limonene), which are not petrochemicals. They are natural fragrance components, and I do not have any sensitivities to them. Even a natural fragrance will drive up a score on an otherwise clean product. It happens often. I have seen it with Dr. Hauschka, a company I love whose products I feel confident in purchasing. Some of their products rank an 8 because of fragrance. I know the company uses essential oils and a natural fragrance formula. However, some essentials oils are toxic and can cause skin allergies and other irritation, while others have more severe side effects. If a company *does not* list the ingredients in the fragrance profile, the ingredient (fragrance or perfume/parfum) will rank an 8. This alone can drive up a product score. If the company *does* list the ingredients, some individual ingredients, such as geraniol or limonene, can rank a moderate to high hazard score.

Greening your beauty routine is not a perfect science, but it's not about being perfect. It's about being informed and knowledgeable. Know your chemicals and decide for yourself what you will and won't allow in your beauty routine. Utilizing the database lets you know exactly where you stand so you can feel confident in your cosmetic selections and be better informed about how to use your 20 percent allowance.

I told you earlier that I was going to let you in on how I keep my favorite products and how you can, too. I use fragrance for my 20 percent chemical allowance. I wear perfume once or twice a month depending on my social activities. Since the rest of my beauty routine is very clean, I can allow for a low-moderate ranking mascara from a company I trust. How do you know you can trust them? Get to know them. Ask yourself these questions:

DO THEY SHARE YOUR VALUES? This is a big one for me. I don't want to purchase products from companies that aren't ethical, compassionate to animals and humans, or sustainable.

DO THEY PROVIDE INGREDIENT LISTS? If they don't provide an ingredient list, it's a problem for me. It doesn't necessarily mean they are hiding something, but I want to know every ingredient in the product *before* I purchase it. This helps me when I shop online and when checking your EWG score. I hate to hunt down ingredient information when I shouldn't have to.

IS THERE TOTAL TRANSPARENCY? I want to know how ingredients are sourced, their business practices, and any social or global humanitarian efforts. If you have trouble finding out information, there is not enough transparency.

DO THEY HAVE ANY CERTIFICATION OR SEALS YOU VALUE? If a company certifies their products USDA Organic, I feel confident that I am getting a quality product. Some standards are stricter than others, so you may have a favorite. I love it when a company is certified cruelty-free and uses the Leaping Bunny logo (refer to Chapter 3 for detailed info on seals and certification).

As you progress on your green beauty journey, you will learn which brands you can trust. Just like knowing the names of chemicals helps you decide how to make chemical allowances, knowing brands and companies' philosophies becomes equally important and comforting. Knowing a company is *certified* natural or organic provides a level of confidence as well.

To determine a score for products that are not in the database, use the Build Your Own Report tool on EWG's website, which you'll find at the top right of the screen. While this may seem complicated, it's actually quite simple. There are four easy steps to customize a report. As an example, here's a report I built from the database by using this tool.

EWG's Skin Deep Cosmetics Database: Build Your Own Report

Sample Product:

W3ll People Bio Extreme Mascara

EWG Score: 3

STEP 1   **Product and Label Information**

First you enter the brand name and product name.
If you do not see it on the drop-down menu, select that
option at the top and add the product name below.

Add the product directions. I selected the "directions not
available" box since the product is mascara and therefore
it is straightforward.

Select the product category from the drop-down menu.
I selected "mascara" for this product and did not add a
second category.

Include claims, indications, or warnings for the product.
I didn't provide any because there were none listed on the
packaging.

Input the ingredients as they appear on the label.
I cut and pasted the ingredients from the W3ll People
website. Nearly all green beauty companies list the
ingredients on the website. If you can't find it on their
website, check other websites that sell the product. Once
you cut and paste the ingredients into the ingredient
window, you can click the "save and continue to step 2"
button at the bottom of the page.

STEP 2   Format the Ingredients for Skin Deep

The database will automatically do this for you, so all you need to do is click "save and continue to step 3."

STEP 3   Ingredients with Skin Deep Matches

If you have any ingredient percentages, add them, and using the drop-down windows, select any listed on the label as qualifying information. I selected "may contain" for the "iron oxides." Proceed to the next step.

STEP 4   View Your Report

Click "View Your Report." The database will break down all the ingredient information for you and give you a score for each ingredient, as well provide any ingredient concerns, including overall hazard, cancer, developmental and reproductive toxicity, allergies and immunotoxicity, and use restrictions.

Report Results:

W3ll People Bio Extreme Mascara

Overall Hazard: LOW-MODERATE

Cancer: LOW

Developmental and reproductive toxicity: LOW

Allergies and immunotoxicity: MODERATE-HIGH

Use restrictions: MODERATE-HIGH

Ingredient Scores:	
Aqua (water)	0
Cera Alba (beeswax)	0
Stearic Acid	1
Copernicia cerifera (carnauba wax)	0
Castor Isostearate beeswax succinate	0
Glyceryl stearate	1
Glycerin	1
Benzyl alcohol	5
Dehydroacetic acid	1
Xanthan gum	0
Cellulose	0
Sodium hydroxide	3
Hydrogenated palm glycerides	0
Tocopherol (vitamin E)	1
Helianthus annuus (sunflower) seed oil	0
Geraniol	7
Limonene	6
Iron oxides (+/-): CI 77499 (iron oxide) (may contain)	2

Now it's your turn. Take your top daily use products and look them up and record their scores using EWG's Skin Deep Cosmetics Database.

Congratulations! You've done the hardest part. You have successfully looked up all your daily use products. Any product higher than a 3 rating should be considered for your 20 percent chemical allowance. If you have a pile that's more than a few products, we've got some work to do to find you alternatives. After you've built your report, you can click on the product tab at the top next to the company name to find clean alternatives. In Day 2, we'll dig a little deeper and evaluate your overall beauty routine and how you can incorporate your favorite products and find alternatives to others to keep you feeling sexy.

DAY 2:
Digging Deeper

WITH YOUR FAVORITE PRODUCTS SET ASIDE, you will now tackle all the remaining products. You don't need a chemistry degree to decode ingredients. Once you adopt the method, you'll be able to read labels in your sleep. Not only will you identify toxic chemicals, you will also begin to identify the safe (or least hazardous) ingredients and their scientific names. You'll also learn how to make all this fit into your life, and what chemicals to allow when.

For example, I like the slip and feel of silicone-based products— a lot. Although there has been concern about silicone as a health hazard, I allow for silicone as an ingredient in hair serums and skin care. Cosmetics-grade silicone is listed as dimethicone, dimethyl polysiloxane, or methicone. It is an effective moisture protector. It is occlusive, which means it creates a barrier on the skin. Because of this, there is concern about its effect as a possible skin allergen and possible organ system toxicant. Dimethicone has an EWG hazard score of 3 out of a possible 10. I don't mind allowing it as an ingredient in my beauty routine from time to time, as long as the rest of the formula is clean and the formula is not a spray. Inhaling a silicone-based product is a health hazard. The idea here is that when you know about the chemical that you are allowing, you can decide when and how to use it.

To do this you need to start getting to know how to identify and ultimately eliminate—and occasionally *allow*—petrochemicals in your beauty routine. If you find that you don't always remember which ingredients are petrochemicals and their risks, the ability to do so will grow over time. To this day, I still look up chemicals I've identified many times before. Don't sweat it. The idea is to start identifying as many toxic chemicals as you can. Also, not all chemicals are bad, which is why I want you to eventually be able to identify them by name. Since not all products are going to be in EWG's database, and you will not always be able to build a report for them when you are shopping, you'll need to "know your stuff" in order to purchase clean products.

SCORE YOUR REMAINING PRODUCTS

Practice with the remaining products you have gathered. Scan the ingredient labels on the ones you use most after your daily use products. Do you see petrochemicals? Remember how to identify them? If not, refer back to Chapter 4. You can look up individual chemicals in the database to find their individual score. In order to determine the toxicity of a product, you may have to make some educated guesses based on what you have learned. It's easy to find a product in the database or build a report on a product, but I want you to look up the chemicals individually. You only need to do a handful of products to start seeing some of the same chemicals over and over again. You will no doubt see parabens and fragrance in addition to FD&C dyes, sodium laureth sulfate, and polyethylene glycol.

Once you begin committing the chemicals to memory, the need to look up the same chemicals will become less frequent. If you need to replace something because you have run out, the product has gone bad, or you need a chemically safe replacement, use the shopping tips in Chapter 6 as a guide or find safe alternatives on EWG's Skin Deep Cosmetics Database just by typing in the product category.

HAVE YOUR ICE-CREAM SUNDAE

Overall, consideration should be given in terms of percentage. For example, let's say you have ten products you use daily. Any one product that scores a 7–10 should be considered as part of your 20 percent allowance. Any two products that score a 4–6 can be considered 20 percent of your allowance. You'll likely have several, and you'll need to find some safer alternatives. It's not precise, but in time you'll intuitively know how clean your daily beauty routine is.

I suggest you replace the products with the highest EWG scores first, but if waste or cash is an issue, replace them as you run out. I have a hard time wasting anything, but this is different. It's up to you to decide when you can replace the products. My job is to help you determine which ones to replace and in what order. The takeaway here is to replace the products that you use most. After several months, you will have many new products in your bags.

Earlier in this chapter, I asked you to set aside your favorite products—your ice-cream sundae (aka "cheat") products. These are the products you'd never dream of parting with. Look them up on the database as well. If they score high enough to warrant replacing (and most likely they will), you can then reassess your attachment. Do you want to make them part of your 20 percent? Could you do without a couple of them for the sake of reducing your chemical exposure? You may be pleasantly surprised. I certainly was when I looked up a traditional eye shadow and found a low EWG score. As a result, I got to keep it and didn't have to use it as part of my 20 percent.

Another and more accurate way to determine your 20 percent is to evaluate the scores of your daily use products. If 80 percent or more score 3 or lower, you are golden. For example, let's use the number ten again. If you use ten products, eight can rate a hazard score of 3 or lower, allowing the remaining two products a higher score. Again, remember, the higher the score, the more weight.

How can you have your ice-cream sundae and eat it too?

1. IDENTIFY YOUR "MUST-HAVE" PRODUCTS. What products make you the happiest or look amazing? Is there a product that is so versatile you can't live without it? Those are your must-haves.

2. SCORE YOUR PRODUCTS ON THE DATABASE. When you look up your products, you know exactly where you stand. You know where to improve and what is already working for you. It will also help you realize what you really want to keep.

3. KNOW WHAT CHEMICALS YOU WILL AND WON'T ALLOW IN YOUR BEAUTY DIET. As you start learning about toxic chemicals, you'll find that you may tolerate some and not others. It will depend on what products you use and value most. For example, I really like a high-performance mascara, so I'll allow a few natural essential oils or natural fragrance chemicals in my mascara. (This can change from day to day and week to week depending on your beauty routine. You may forgo your daily cheat products on the week you get your hair colored or wear fragrance, such as I do.)

4. DECIDE HOW YOU WILL USE YOUR 20 PERCENT CHEMICAL ALLOWANCE (YOUR ICE-CREAM SUNDAE). Now that you know your must-have products and your scores, try to create an 80/20 balance in your daily routine.

A Peek Inside My Personal Makeup Kit

W3LL PEOPLE EXPRESSIONIST BIO EXTREME MASCARA BLACK (EWG score: 3): Gives me long, lush lashes without feeling stiff.

VAPOUR ORGANIC BEAUTY ATMOSPHERE LUMINOUS FOUNDATION (EWG score: 2): Blends easily and feels light on my skin.

W3LL PEOPLE COLORBALM, NUDIST NO 6 (EWG score: 3*): I love the sheer chocolate color and balm combo.

ZUII ORGANIC CERTIFIED ORGANIC FLORA FOUNDATION, ALMOND (EWG score: 1*): Warms up my skin without depositing too much pigment.

JANE IREDALE JUST KISSED LIP AND CHEEK, SAMPLE SIZE (EWG score: 1*): I rub this on my cheeks and lips for a quick bit of color. The glossy texture is gorg.

PACIFICA EYELINER SMOLDER EYE LINING GEL, MIDNIGHT (EWG score: 2*): A fabulous blue-black color for day-to-night transitions.

JANE IREDALE IN TOUCH HIGHLIGHTER (EWG score: 2): Silky smooth and hydrating, and not too shimmery.

BEAUTYCOUNTER TOUCHUP SKIN CONCEALER PEN (EWG score: 1): A brilliant quick fix for under eyes.

BEAUTYCOUNTER COLOR DEFINE BROW PENCIL (EWG score: 0): Blends seamlessly with my brows and stays on all day.

ANTONYM CERTIFIED ORGANIC EYELINER PENCIL (EWG score: 2*): The deep black defines gorgeously and is soft enough for my waterline and smudging.

Throughout the book, an asterisk (*) following the EWG score indicates that the product is not in the EWG Skin Deep Cosmetics Database and that the score is based on EWG's Build Your Own Report tool.

You can do this. What's more, you will enjoy doing this because it will allow you to feel empowered and confident while shopping for new cosmetics. You will want to give up products and seek out healthy alternatives. After all, who doesn't want to buy new makeup? This is a great excuse to splurge on a few new products or try a new eye shadow color or foundation. Go ahead! Purge, then splurge!

Chapter Six

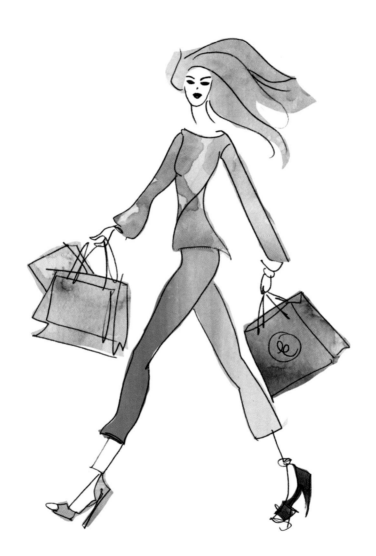

SHOP like a

Pro!

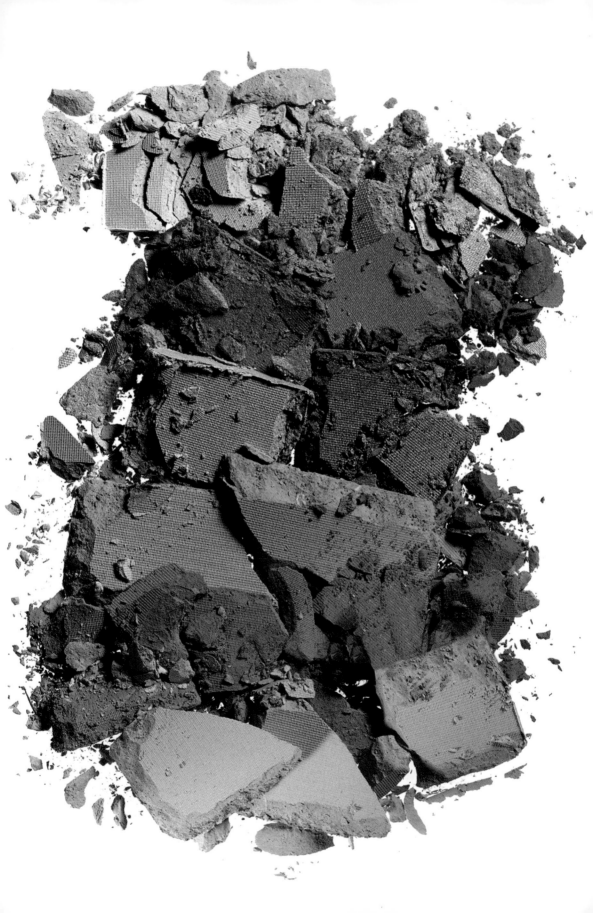

This is where the real fun begins. It's all about shopping. You'll be able to shop for products in department stores, drugstores, health food stores, and online. You will be so prepared that you'll be able to walk into any retail outlet and select products with confidence. As an advocate for the consumer, I want to help you navigate the daunting green shopping experience and find chemically safe, quality products.

By now you know what you're looking for in terms of which chemicals to avoid and which to allow. When you're not able to rank a product using the database, your aim is to eliminate as many toxic ingredients and petrochemicals as possible without having to eliminate a large number of products that are absolutely safe to use. Be as discriminating as possible, unless you have something very specific in mind or you are in a place, such as an airport or desolate area, where it is difficult to find clean, natural, and eco-friendly products. Remember the eco-attitudes in Chapter 1? This is where they'll come in handy.

Drugstore Superstars

1. **EGYPTIAN MAGIC** (EWG score: 0)

2. **PHYSICIANS FORMULA** Organic Wear Bronzer (EWG score: 2)

3. BURT'S BEES Lip Crayon (EWG score: 2*)

4. EOS lip balm (EWG score: 1)

5. ALBA BOTANICA HAWAIIAN EYE GEL (EWG score: 2)

6. AVALON ORGANICS CoQ10 Repair Wrinkle Defense Cream (EWG score: 2)

7. SHEA Moisture African Black Soap (EWG score: 2*)

8. NATURE'S GATE Cleansing Milk Normal/Dry Skin, Rice Bran (EWG score: 2)

9. DR. BRONNER'S MAGIC SOAPS 18-in-1 Hemp Pure-Castile Soap, Peppermint (EWG score: 1)

10. DESERT ESSENCE Tea Tree Oil and Neem Toothpaste (EWG score: 1)

11. DICKINSON'S Daily Facial Towelettes (EWG score: 1)

12. MYCHELLE DERMACEUTICALS Supreme Polypeptide Cream Age Defense (Unscented) (EWG score: 1*)

13. DERMA *e* Age-Defying Antioxidant Eye Crème (EWG score: 2)

14. PHYSICIANS FORMULA Organic Wear 100% Natural Origin Mascara, Ultra Black (EWG score: 1)

15. ECOTOOLS Bamboo 5 piece Brush Set (no score)

16. EMANI VEGAN Cosmetics Perfect 10 Primer Serum (EWG score: 2)

17. OUT OF AFRICA 100% Pure & Unrefined Shea Butter Tin, Vanilla/Unscented (EWG score: 0)

18. AUBREY ORGANICS Natural Sun Sport Stick Sunscreen, SPF 30+ (EWG score: 1)

19. ANDALOU NATURALS CC 1000 Roses Color + Correct (EWG score: 1)

20. SEED HEALTHY HAND CREAM (EWG score: 1)

DRUGSTORES AND BIG BOX STORES: RESEARCH IN ADVANCE

1. CHECK THE STORE'S WEBSITE. Websites often have a green, natural, or organic cosmetic category. If not, check out their brands.

2. DO YOUR DUE DILIGENCE. Check brand websites. Once you find brands that look chemically safe, you can check out their websites for a deeper look. Read their mission statements and philosophy. Companies who wax on about their mission are usually the real deal, or at least they're trying. Dr. Bronner's soaps are a good example of this. You should be able to find out if they are chemically safe with just a few clicks.

Remember my three favorite online resources: Campaign for Safe Cosmetics (*safecosmetics.org*), EWG's Skin Deep Cosmetics Database (*http://www.ewg.org/skindeep/*), and Women's Voices for the Earth (*http://www.womensvoices.org/*).

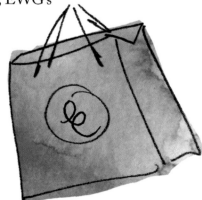

SIXTY-SECOND SAVE

I have a technique I use when shopping for natural and organic products when I haven't done any prior research on the brand or stores. It comes in handy when I am unexpectedly shopping, which is often. It's supereasy and incorporates everything you have already learned.

1. **SCAN FOR SEALS/CERTIFICATIONS.** First, look for the seals I mention in Chapter 3. It's the easiest way to locate a clean product. But as you know, criteria are different for each certification and some are stricter than others. Next, don't scan for just any green marketing. Look for specific words, especially those products that say they are free of parabens, synthetic dyes, fragrance, and petrochemicals.

2. **LOOK FOR GREEN MARKETING.** Look for packaging that advertises the products as chemically safe/green. Companies who are the real deal generally incorporate it into their marketing. The more specific the better. The words "natural" and "organic" are not enough. However "free of parabens, synthetics, talc, SLS, and petrochemicals" would be a brand I would investigate further. There are tons of amazing chemically safe and natural products that are *not* certified, so don't be afraid if you don't see a seal on a product that otherwise checks out to be chemically safe.

3. **BE A "BOX TURNER."** Flip over the box and examine the ingredients. It is necessary to check every box to be certain you are getting a quality product. It should be the first step before buying a product. You know how to read the label:

   Look for the Three Ps and identify the potentially toxic chemicals, if any.

Check to see where potentially toxic or unknown ingredients fall in the list/label.

You have the skills you need to make smart choices. You can always try scanning the product on your Skin Deep Cosmetics Database app (*http://www.ewg.org/skindeep/*) if you need some help. By now you already know so much, you should feel confident to make choices on your own.

DEPARTMENT STORES AND HEALTH FOOD STORES

In department stores and health food stores, you will get more personalized service and experienced sales associates. The salespeople are trained with the products or generally know much more about them than a drugstore or big box store sales associate would. I have seen this change a bit with some stores, such as CVS and Target, where they have a person designated to the cosmetics area, but I have not found them that knowledgeable about green products. You will likely know more than they do at this point. That must feel good! Here is how I approach shopping in department stores:

1. **GET HELP:** Ask the salesperson if there are any natural or organic brands. They will have several to offer, but not all are as clean as the sales associates are trained to believe. They are not experts on chemically safe products, so you have to be. They will know which ones are touting themselves as green but often not much more in terms of how safe it really is. They are, however, well trained with the products and can tell you how to use them and get the best results. Ask the

associates for more information or literature on the company or product and always ask for samples. We love samples.

2. **CONTACT THE COMPANY:** Don't be afraid to e-mail or call the cosmetic companies with questions. I routinely ask about fragrance. Express your concerns, ask questions, or request a sample be mailed to you. Often you will be paying a lot more in these stores since they carry premium products. Make sure it's something you feel is worth it.

ONLINE SHOPPING

Be Social

After you've done the initial research and identified companies or products that are green, take it to social media. There are several ways in which social media can help you know what you are getting. Reach out on Twitter, Facebook, or Instagram. Ask your followers or friends for their input. Today I sent out a tweet asking if anyone had tried Iba Halal products. It's a new company based in India, but they are selling their products in the United States and the United Kingdom, and I wanted to get some feedback before I made an investment, or phone call, in my case.

Read Reviews

Check out product reviews. I usually do a search for reviews on Google using the product name, but any search engine will do. Be sure to check the company website for reviews as well. And while you are there, read the product descriptions. They know their products best. It's not unusual for a company to tell you how to use a product or which skin type it will work best on. Pay special attention to the color descriptions; they will tell you more than looking at the swatch.

Also, read reviews on other retailer and beauty websites, such as amazon.com, drugstore.com and totalbeauty.com. Online boutiques stores will often have them, too. Lastly, check the reference section for a list of my favorite green beauty bloggers.

Nearly every online store has added the social media element to the experience. Occasionally, there aren't any reviews. When that happens, I check other product reviews from the same company. I find that when a company has many stellar products, my chances are good that it will be good quality, if not a hero product.

Here are some things to look for on the reviews:

1. COLOR/TEXTURE/SMELL: You can't tell a color from the swatch online. They are never accurate in my experience. Companies will usually give you a description, and that helps, but pay attention to the reviews more. Patrons will tell you in what way the color differs from the swatch or describe it more accurately. It may be as simple as, "it's more of a red than a pink," or "it looks pink on the swatch but when I tried it on, it looked redder." Sometimes it's more complicated and you see things like, "it was true beige when I first applied the lipstick but after a couple of hours, it went orange." Listen to the reviewers. The information is invaluable. I have learned the hard way that if enough reviews say the same thing, it's probably going to be true for me as well.

2. CUSTOMER SERVICE: In addition to getting a superior product, I care about customer service. Reviewers will say when a product took way too long to arrive or arrived in bad condition. Were they able to get a replacement product without any hassle? Did people have a hard time returning products?

People will call out poor customer service. If enough people are saying their customer service is bad, it's probably true. I bought a headboard for my bed while traveling on the road. Online shopping is how I killed time on the tour bus. The headboard arrived while I was away, but by then I had found another one online that I liked more. When I finally got home, it had been several weeks until I could get around to returning it, but the company took it back graciously without any problem, and they even paid for the shipping, which was more than $100. I shop there as much as possible now, and their customer service is always excellent. I won't shop at stores that do not have exceptional customer service.

3. USE SUGGESTIONS: Reviewers aren't shy about telling you how they use a product or what to do to get it to perform its best. They'll give you good insight on how much you will need to work with a product, if at all. Not only that, they will tell you what they paired it with and how to layer it.

4. PRODUCT RECOMMENDATIONS: If a person recommends another product, check it out. When a person raves about more than one product from the same company, they may be onto something good.

BE A SUPER SLEUTH

M essage boards on green beauty sites are candy stores for information about eco-friendly beauty products. Read the blogs as well as the comments and forums.

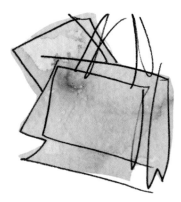

Shop These Online Stores

AMAZON *(www.amazon.com)* The granddaddy of online shopping. You can find just about any chemically safe beauty product you need. If you have a Prime membership, you'll save money on shipping.

BEAUTORIUM *(http://www.beautorium.com/)* This website offers beauty products from boutique brands like Revolution Organics, Kimberly Sayer, and Indie Lee. The ability to shop by beauty issues such as blemished or sensitive skin takes out some of the guess work.

CREDO BEAUTY *(credobeauty.com)* A cool website that integrates maker videos, Instagram, and a blog. When you order from their extensive collection of boutique (and some mass) brands you get samples in every order. Love that!

GREEN LINE BEAUTY *(www.greenlinebeauty.com)* I love the tightly edited selection of high quality chemically safe products. One of the purest, most luxurious skin care selections from brands such as Sodashi and Dr. Alkaitis.

DRUGSTORE.COM AND BEAUTY.COM *(http://www.drugstore .com/)* The site hosts a large variety of green drugstore brands across all categories, such as Burt's Bees and Alba Botanica, with excellent prices and helpful reviews.

LUCKY VITAMIN *(www.luckyvitamin.com)* A healthy lifestyle store with a large selection of green beauty products. What's great about it is that you can shop by specialty, such as vegan, organic, non-GMO.

PHARMACA *(www.pharmaca.com)* A terrific integrative pharmacy with an large range of color cosmetics and a nice selection of affordable natural fragrances including Love & Toast and Pacifica.

SPIRIT BEAUTY LOUNGE *(http://www.spiritbeautylounge.com/)* They offer a beautifully curated selection of premium products, such as Kjaer Weis, May Lindstrom Skin, and Strange Invisible Perfumes, as well as expert picks.

THE DETOX MARKET *(www.thedetoxmarket.com)* An impressive selection of cosmetics across all categories. The makeup collection stands out for being well rounded and gorgeous.

THRIVE MARKET *(thrivemarket.com)* An online shopping club that is bringing organics to the masses. Their small but growing beauty section is worth the wait at 25 to 50 percent off retail prices. Plus, you can shop by values such as Vegan, Gluten-free, and Healthy Moms.

VITACOST *(www.vitacost.com)* A healthy lifestyle store that has a decent selection of mass green beauty brands. With great prices and a 100 percent money-back guarantee, it's a great place to try new products.

NICHE SHOPPING: VEGAN AND GLUTEN-FREE BEAUTY

To help you get started with your vegan and gluten-free cosmetics I am providing you with a small selection of cosmetic brands that offer these types of products. In the Resources section in the back of the book I list many of my favorite brands. Be sure to check their websites for vegan and gluten-free cosmetics as I have certainly not listed them all.

Vegan Cosmetic Brands

100% PURE: A majority of the products are vegan with the exception of a few products that contain beeswax, goat's milk, cruelty-free honey, and pearl powder.

AFTERGLOW COSMETICS: The majority of their products are vegan. They use beeswax in a few of their lip and eye products. Check the website for a list.

BEAUTY WITHOUT CRUELTY: 100 percent vegan.

DERMA *e*: 100 percent vegan.

DESERT ESSENCE: 100 percent vegan.

ECCO BELLA: A majority of their products are vegan. Only a small selection of makeup uses carmine as a colorant. Skin care is vegan.

EMANI: 100 percent vegan.

GABRIEL COSMETICS: 100 percent vegan.

HUGO NATURALS: 100 percent vegan.

HYNT BEAUTY: 100 percent vegan.

INIKA: 100 percent vegan.

JANE IREDALE: This company has some vegan products. Check the website for a list of products that are *not* vegan.

ZUZU LUXE: 100 percent vegan.

GLUTEN-FREE BRANDS

100% PURE: Most of their products are gluten-free, with the exception of their mascaras.

AFTERGLOW COSMETICS: 100 percent gluten-free.

DERMA *e*: 100 percent gluten-free.

ECCO BELLA: 100 percent gluten-free.

HUGO NATURALS: Gluten-free, except for the Shea Butter & Oatmeal Bar Soap and the Oatmeal Mint Artisan-Bulk Soap.

JANE IREDALE: Most products are gluten-free. Check their website for a list of products that are *not* gluten-free.

JUICE BEAUTY: 100 percent gluten-free.

LAVERA: 100 percent gluten-free.

RMS BEAUTY: These products are gluten-free with the exception of the mascara.

ZUII ORGANIC: 100 percent gluten-free.

ZUZU LUXE: 100 percent gluten-free.

You've just learned all my favorite stores, my most clever shopping strategies, and my best shopping tips. You will be able to replace your high-scoring products without having to sleuth out the stores. No more trolling endless beauty aisles for just one clean brand or spending a small fortune on a green beauty fake. Now give yourself permission to splurge on a green beauty shopping spree. You're worth it!

Fabulous Finds for $15 and Under

GABRIEL EYE SHADOW (EWG score: 2): The velvety matte finish gives you a natural look.

GIOVANNI HOT CHOCOLATE SUGAR SCRUB (EWG score: 2): Your man will go bananas for this sweet-smelling exfoliant that leaves your skin silky smooth.

JANE IREDALE 24-KARAT GOLD DUST (EWG score: 2): A soft, iridescent eye shadow that looks gorgeous alone or layered over eye shadow.

JOHN MASTERS ORGANICS BARE UNSCENTED SHAMPOO (EWG score: 2): Ideal for those sensitive to fragrance.

JUICE BEAUTY GREEN APPLE AGE DEFY HAND CREAM (EWG score: 2*): A fast-absorbing cream that keeps your hands looking as young as your face.

LE COUVENT DES MINIMES SMILE LIP BALM VERY RICH FORMULA HONEY AROMA (EWG score: 0*) This lip balm provides a rich intense hydration. Works well as a lip mask too.

MINERAL FUSION SHEER MOISTURE LIP TINTS (EWG score: 2): Subtle shine and color payoff; it's the perfect sheer lip tint.

SCOTCH NATURALS LACQUER, NEAT (EWG score: 1): Make your boss jealous with this "all free" perfect neutral pink.

TATCHA ABURATORIGAMI JAPANESE BEAUTY PAPERS (no score): These facial blotting papers are wonderful to have in your purse, carry on or car. I often prefer these to powder.

ZUZU LUXE CREAM BROW PENCIL (EWG score: 2): A long lasting brow pencil that glides on and stays put.

Toss & Try: Green Beauty Swaps

TOSS: Yves Saint Laurent Touche Éclat Radiant Touch

TRY: Beautycounter Touchup Skin Concealer Pen (EWG score: 1)

TOSS: Nars Blush in Orgasm

TRY: Zuii Organic Certified Organic Flora Blush in Melon (EWG score: 2*)

TOSS: Nars Copacabana The Multiple

TRY: RMS Beauty Living Luminizer (EWG score: 1)

TOSS: Chanel Le Vernis in Black Satin

TRY: Deborah Lippmann Nail Color Fade to Black (EWG score: 2*)

TOSS: M.A.C. Lipstick in Russian Red

TRY: Ilia Lipstick Strike It Up (EWG score: 2*)

TOSS: Makeup Forever High Definition Powder

TRY: W3ll People Realist Invisible Setting Powder (EWG score: 1*)

TOSS: Chanel Crayon Sourcils Sculpting Eyebrow Pencil

TRY: Beautycounter Color Define Brow Pencil (EWG score: 1)

TOSS: Bobbi Brown Long-Wear Cream Shadow

TRY: 100% Pure Fruit Pigmented Satin Eye Shadow (EWG score: 1*)

TOSS: Laura Mercier Secret Camouflage

TRY: Jane Iredale Circle Delete Concealer (EWG score: 2)

TOSS: Revlon Just Bitten Kissable Balm Stain

TRY: 100% Pure Lip Tint (EWG score: 2*)

Chapter Seven

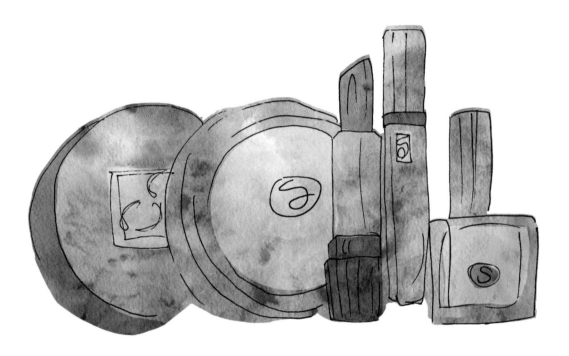

The **GREEN** Beauty *Kit*

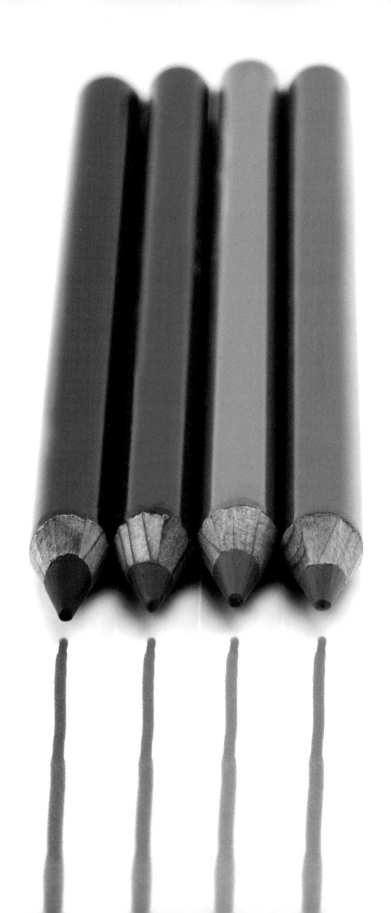

You didn't think I would tell you all about those dirty toxins and not give you some fabulous beauty referrals, did you? Not a chance! I am thrilled to open my personal and professional beauty kits to you and reveal my favorite green beauty products. I'm sharing all my star products for every budget, removing the guesswork and the trial and error of shopping for chemically safe, natural, and organic products that work. I have looked up each product to bring you only the cleanest high-performance beauty products.

All the products I am sharing are not only my favorites but they score a 3 or lower in the EWG's Skin Deep Cosmetics Database, with the vast majority of the products scoring a 2 or lower. As you may have figured out by scoring your own products, it's extremely difficult to find products that rank a 2 or lower on the EWG Cosmetics Database. I worked hard to compile a list of the highest-performing and lowest-scoring products. Use this list to assemble the core body of clean beauty products for your daily routine while still keeping the products that you love and that make you feel beautiful.

As you learn more, you will naturally find products you love along the way, but this will get you started. If you are not quite ready for such a big transition, these beauty products can be used as alternatives to the traditional products that you are ready to replace. That's why I mostly recommended products that score only a 2 or lower, so you have a lot of room to play.

There are many wonderful, natural, and chemically safe cosmetic companies and products that I love and use that I did not mention in the book because their products score above a 3. This doesn't mean that they aren't quality or all-natural. It simply means that some of the ingredients—natural or otherwise—ranked too high. In some instances, it's because the formula doesn't have all the ingredients properly specified to get the most accurate score. For example, Ecco Bella's products rank higher because they list flower waxes as an ingredient. Because each flower wax is not specified individually, the database ranks "unspecified waxes" as a 4 because not all flower waxes are the same and the EWG values transparency. I know Ecco Bella's values and they are among the highest but the database will always rank a higher score when waxes and oils are not individually specified. You can see below that the 4 drives up the score, since all the other ingredients score 0–2. I love Ecco Bella's values and trust their formulas. Here is an example of an ingredients list from an Ecco Bella product:

Ecco Bella FlowerColor Cover Up Ingredients List	
Castor oil	EWG score: 2
Isopropyl palmitate *(from palm oil)*	EWG score: 0
Candelilla wax	EWG score: 0
Beeswax	EWG score: 1
Organic calendula oil	EWG score: 1
Organic chamomile oil	EWG score: 1
Organic jojoba oil	EWG score: 1
100 iu vitamin E	EWG score: 1
Titanium dioxide	EWG score: 1
Flower wax	EWG score: 4
Iron oxides	EWG score: 2

In other cases, such as Dr. Hauschka, Intelligent Nutrients, Amala, and many other natural and organic cosmetic companies, the word "fragrance" or "aroma" have driven up the score. Even though the label states that the fragrance is derived from natural essential oils, the database will pick up the word "fragrance," "aroma," and "essential oils" and compute the score higher. There are a few naturally occurring scent ingredients that are very popular among green cosmetic companies that will make a score higher, such as geraniol, eugenol, coumarin, and limonene, to name a few. While they are all components of natural fragrance they are considered allergens and/or irritants and will be ranked accordingly. Other companies that use vitamin A derivatives will also score higher since these ingredients score a 9 on the database. ZuZu Luxe is one company that formulates with retinyl palmitate. I love their products and use them regularly. While I have not included these products because they ranked higher than a 3, I use products from each of these companies, and others not mentioned. I am comfortable with these naturally occurring fragrance components and vitamin A derivatives (especially retinyl palimitate, which is not as strong as retinol) but I excluded these products from the list to help you find the cleanest, most nonirritating products possible. However, I would absolutely refer them to friends or clients.

We all have different criteria for our chemical allowance. I want you to be able to decide if you will allow these natural fragrance components or vitamin A derivatives. If so, then I have listed many of these companies in the Resources section in the back of the book and on my website where I list them and have blogged about these products. You can always check out paigepadgett.com for more product referrals in addition to connecting with me on social media. All my user names are Paige Padgett, so it's easy to find me. I am always giving product referrals on Twitter, Facebook, Pinterest, and Instagram.

It's up to you to decide what chemicals you will or won't allow in your green beauty diet. At times you may feel fine with a particular chemical while other times you won't.

I am not fanatical at all about my products. If you have a core body of ultraclean products, you don't have to sweat the small stuff, the one-offs, special-occasion, use-it-on-the-tips-of-your-hair products. I make sure my day-to-day core products are superclean so I have lots of room to play with other natural products that may score higher. You may feel that anything that is natural is fine, high score or otherwise. Still, I thought it would be best for me to give you only the products with scores of 3 or lower. I'll leave it up to you to decide which products to use that score higher.

PRIMER

HYNT BEAUTY RADIANCE BOOSTER (EWG score: 2*): A wonderful skin prep that leaves your skin so gorgeous you may not want to cover up with foundation.

ZUII ORGANIC CERTIFIED ORGANIC FOUNDATION PRIMER (EWG score: 1*): A refreshing lightweight formula that soothes and calms the skin while providing a bit of oil control.

JANE IREDALE ABSENCE OIL CONTROL PRIMER (EWG score: 2*): Controls oil like a champ. A little goes a long way, so apply only where needed.

TARTE CLEAN SLATE 12-HOUR PERFECTING PRIMER (EWG score: 2): Creates a flawless finish by greatly minimizing pores. Pair with concealer only for a natural finish.

FOUNDATION

Stick/Pan

W3LL PEOPLE NARCISSIST FOUNDATION CONCEALER (EWG score: 2): A great multitasking stick foundation that doubles as a concealer and provides a flawless finish. A must-have for your carry-on.

KJAER WEIS FOUNDATION (EWG score: 1*): Pan makeup that blends easily and sheers out to a velvety matte finish.

VAPOUR ORGANIC BEAUTY ATMOSPHERE LUMINOUS FOUNDATION (EWG score: 2): A beautiful, sheer coverage that melts into the skin. It's silky enough to use under the eyes too.

Liquid

ZUZU LUXE OIL FREE LIQUID FOUNDATION (EWG score: 3): I was drawn to this liquid foundation for its wide range of colors, but I stayed for its silky finish.

KOH GEN DO MAIFANSHI MOISTURE FOUNDATION (EWG score: 2*): I love this foundation for its hydrating, flawless finish.

JANE IREDALE LIQUID MINERALS FOUNDATION (EWG score: 2): This provides a natural-looking, medium coverage that works well on all skin types. Use a fluffy foundation brush to break up the minerals.

Pressed Powder Foundation

ZUII ORGANIC CERTIFIED ORGANIC FLORA FOUNDATION (EWG score: 1*): A natural-looking, medium coverage pressed-powder foundation that doesn't look chalky or ashy. Works well as a setting powder too.

JANE IREDALE PUREPRESSED BASE MINERAL FOUNDATION (EWG score: 2): A highly pigmented, full-coverage powder that's ideal for when you want a superpolished look.

EMANI FLAWLESS MATTE FOUNDATION (EWG score: 2*): Creates a medium matte finish that looks natural, not cakey.

BRIGHTENING/FINISHING POWDER

W3LL PEOPLE REALIST INVISIBLE SETTING POWDER (EWG score: 1*): Like a magical dust, it leaves you with an airbrushed look. Yes, please!

GLAMNATURAL FINISHING POWDER (EWG score: 0*): Takes down shine and leaves a dewy finish. It's not too matte.

HYNT BEAUTY FINALE FINISHING POWDER (EWG score: 1*): Sets makeup beautifully with a light finish that's not ashy on darker skin tones.

BB CREAM/TINTED MOISTURIZER

BEAUTYCOUNTER SKIN TINT (EWG score: 2*): Superemollient with just the right amount of color. The perfect tinted moisturizer.

JANE IREDALE GLOW TIME FULL COVERAGE BB CREAM (EWG score: 1): The multitasking benefits of a BB cream with the coverage of a foundation. Ideal for those seeking to minimize their daily routine.

SUNTEGRITY SKINCARE 5 IN 1 NATURAL MOISTURIZING FACE BROAD SPECTRUM SUNSCREEN (EWG score: 1): Another amazing multitasker. I love this sunscreen so much for its coverage and finish that I categorized it as a BB cream rather than a sunscreen.

CONCEALER

BEAUTYCOUNTER TOUCHUP SKIN CONCEALER PEN (EWG score: 1): A generous amount of pigment qualifies it as a cover-up, but what I think is so great is the peachy undertones that make it more like a corrector that brightens the eyes.

RMS BEAUTY "UN" COVER-UP (EWG score: 1): One of my all-time favorites. Dewy enough for under the eyes but enough coverage for a blemish. Perfection.

HYNT BEAUTY DUO PHASE HYDRATING CONCEALER (EWG score: 2*): A heavy-duty concealer that conceals even the worst skin problems.

MINERAL FUSION CONCEALER DUO, NEUTRAL (EWG score: 2): A good lightweight concealer for under eyes. Blend the colors to conceal with perfect perfection.

LIPSTICK

ILIA LIPSTICK (EWG score: 2*): Light and moisturizing yet packs a punch of pigment.

ZUII ORGANIC CERTIFIED ORGANIC FLORA LIPSTICK (EWG score: 2*): Long-lasting and hydrating with vitamins A, C, and E.

ECCO BELLA FLOWERCOLOR LIPSTICK (EWG score: 3): Rich colors and texture make this lipstick wear beautifully.

Lip Tint/Sheer

BEAUTYCOUNTER COLOR LIP SHEER (EWG score: 1): Provides sheer color with a pretty shine. Highly versatile for a variety of beauty looks.

ALIMA PURE LIP TINTS (EWG score: 2): Packs more pigment that many balm tints. Smells and tastes great.

W3LL PEOPLE (EWG score: 3): Great for multitasking, it's a balm and a lipstick in one.

Lip Gloss

JANE IREDALE PURE LIP GLOSS (EWG score: 1): It's hard to find amazing chemically safe gloss, but this formula is so good. High shine and not goopy. Pink Smoothie is my fave.

EMANI ORGANIC LIP SHINE, BLUSH (EWG score: 2*): Gorgeous color saturation and long-lasting shine make this gloss a must-have for every kit.

100% PURE FRUIT PIGMENTED LIP GLOSS, SHEER STRAWBERRY (EWG score: 1*): I love the perfect mix of creamy neutral and sheer bright color selection sans all the shimmer.

EYE SHADOWS

Powder

GLAMNATURAL EYESHADOW, COCOA MAUVE (EWG score: 2*): One of the silkiest eye shadows I've used. It practically glides on by itself.

BEAUTYCOUNTER COLOR SHADE EYE DUO, SHELL/MALT (EWG score: 1): Perfectly paired colors to use together or alone.

ZUZU LUXE EYESHADOW (EWG score: 2): A long-wearing gorgeous range of matte and luminous textures in the prettiest colors.

Cream/Liquid

JANE IREDALE EYE GLOSS LIQUID EYE SHADOW (EWG score: 1): One of the most under-the-radar eye shadows ever. Not really a gloss, it dries down like a watercolor to create the prettiest eyes.

100% PURE FRUIT PIGMENTED SATIN EYE SHADOW, BORA BORA (EWG score: 1*): Goes on smooth and creamy but doesn't crease. Great for sensitive eyes.

VAPOUR ORGANIC MESMERIZE EYE COLOR (EWG score: 1): Soft, sheer color gives this shadow a pretty, natural look.

EYELINER

Pencil

MINERAL FUSION EYE PENCIL (EWG score: 1): A silky-soft pencil that glides on easily and doesn't irritate the eyes.

ZUZU LUXE EYE LINER PENCIL (EWG score: 2): A long lasting pencil that has pretty green and blue color options.

100% PURE FRUIT PIGMENTED CREAM STICK EYE LINER, BLACK-BERRY (EWG score: 1*): I love this creamy, chubby liner for creating smudgy, smoky eyes without any eye shadow.

Liquid

JANE IREDALE LIQUID LINER (EWG score: 1): I love the way it dries down to a matte finish.

ZUZU LUXE LIQUID EYELINER (EWG score: 3): What's great about this is the precision sponge-tipped wand. Makes the novice look like a pro.

100% PURE BLACK TEA LONG LAST LIQUID EYE LINER (EWG score: 0*): The fine brush allows you to make the tightest lines to gorgeously define your eyes.

Gel

JANE IREDALE JELLY JAR (EWG score: 1): An easy to maneuver inky gel liner that wears well—no smearing.

PACIFICA SMOLDER EYE LINING GEL (EWG score: 2*): Creamy enough to smudge or leave sharp. Midnight is my favorite color.

TARTE CLAY POT AMAZONIAN CLAY WATERPROOF LINER (EWG score: 2): Bold colors that go on smoothly and don't transfer.

BROW COLOR

BEAUTYCOUNTER COLOR DEFINE BROW PENCIL (EWG score: 0): The perfect dual-ended spoolie and brow pencil, this formula rivals all the premium brands.

ECOBROW (EWG score: 3*): Buildable wax and natural colors make it easy to create full brows. Has a celebrity cult following.

ZUII ORGANICS BROW DEFINER (EWG score: 1): The design is genius. It's like having a pencil and an angle brush all in one. The texture isn't too matte; it looks more like skin.

MASCARA

ANTONYM LOLA LASHES (EWG score: 2): Certified natural mascara, deeply black and super buildable.

W3LL PEOPLE BIO EXTREME MASCARA (EWG score: 3): A lengthening and volumizing mascara that will make you forget everything you ever thought about natural mascara. It's that good.

100% PURE BLACK TEA PIGMENTED ULTRA LENGTHENING MASCARA (EWG score: 2): A soft, buildable mascara with a fruity smell. The purple is my favorite.

BLUSH

BEAUTYCOUNTER SWEEP BLUSH DUO, TAWNY WHISPER (EWG score: 1*): I love the two-tone colors. It takes all the guesswork out of creating sculpted cheekbones.

ZUII ORGANIC CERTIFIED ORGANIC FLORA BLUSH, MELON (EWG score: 2*): This pink-gold blush is gorgeous on all skin tones. This luminous blush provides a healthy flush.

ECCO BELLA FLOWERCOLOR BLUSH, CORAL ROSE (EWG score: 2*): Lots of pigment payoff in pretty matte colors.

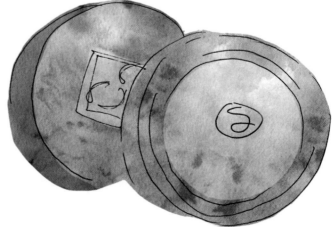

HIGHLIGHTER

RMS BEAUTY LIVING LUMINIZER (EWG score: 1): This lives up to all the hype. It beautifully illuminizes the skin with a dewy finish.

KJAER WEISS LUMINIZER RADIANCE (EWG score: 2*): Wear this on top of your lids paired with mascara, or pop your cheekbones with this warm, summery pearl highlighter.

INIKA LIGHT REFLECT HIGHLIGHTING CRÈME (EWG score: 1): This creamy hydrating luminizer is so versatile. Mix it in your foundation or moisturizer for all-over illumination or highlight your cheekbones and brow bone.

BRONZER

W3LL PEOPLE BIO BRONZER NATURAL TAN (EWG score: 1*): I like this because it reminds me of my first bronzer—Indian Earth. This has that same sexy, desert, sun-kissed look.

COULEUR CARAMEL BRONZER (EWG score: 1*): A fabulous baked bronzer that you'll want to use as a contour too.

ZUZU LUXE BRONZER (EWG score: 2): I love this bronzer with illuminization. It's not too shimmery. It's just so gorgeous.

MULTITASKING PRODUCTS

JANE IREDALE JUST KISSED LIP AND CHEEK STAIN (EWG score: 1*): Brighten your look with a swipe of this across your lips and cheeks. Provides a dewy look.

W3LL PEOPLE UNIVERSALIST MULTI-USE COLOR STICK, NO. 8
(EWG score: 2*): The satiny smooth finish and high pigment payoff makes this ideal for eye, lips, and cheeks.

GABRIEL COSMETICS MULTI POT, PINK PETAL (EWG score: 2*): A multi pot that works well on eyes, cheeks and lips with a waxy powder finish. Apply lip balm before using on your lips for a hydrated smooth finish.

TOOLS

ARTIS MAKEUP BRUSHES: I love these brushes. They feel amazing on the skin and blend makeup beautifully. You would never know they are made with synthetic bristles.

SONIA KASHUK: Sonia offers a wide range of stylish brush kits at affordable prices

ECOTOOLS: One of my all-time favorites for eco-friendliness and affordability. Plus, they do the best kits.

TARTE: These brushes are great quality and work so well. I love the foundation brush and stipple brush.

BEAUTY BLENDER: A good makeup sponge to use wet or dry. Blend foundation seamlessly with a slight roll of the wrist.

TWEEZERMAN: Tweezerman not only has the best selection of top-notch tweezers, they also have other handy facial grooming tools.

CLARISONIC: Manually exfoliates dead skin. My skin glows after I use it.

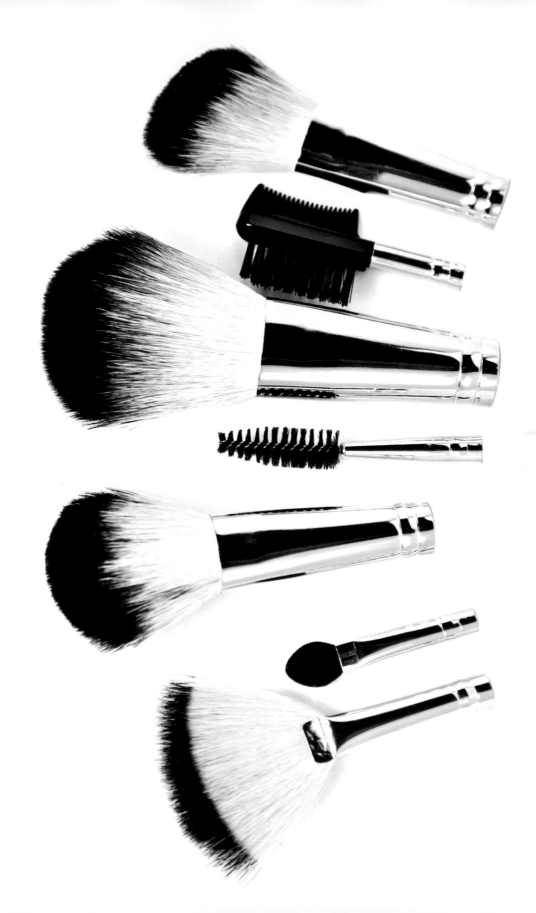

Paige's Top Ten Tools

Nothing can stop me dead in my tracks like not being able to find my brushes. I've stormed through airports, run after cabs, and torn my house to pieces just to make sure they're safe and sound. For me, my brushes mean business. For you, they should mean pleasure. Tools of the beauty trade and good supplies can be the difference between tantalizing and terrible. These are the brushes I can't live without:

1. **EYESHADOW SHADER** brush has a small, flat, stiff brush to deposit pigment to the eyelid. Good for shading the crease or smudging the lash line.

2. **SOFT DOME BLENDER BRUSH** works well to disperse a wash of color and for blending and hard edges.

3. **LARGE, FLUFFY, SOFT SHADOW BRUSH** is perfect for powdering small areas or highlighter and applying a wash of color.

4. **ANGLED LINER BRUSH** is the most user-friendly for a precise line. Doubles as an eyebrow brush.

5. **FLUFFY FLAT OR STIPPLE FOUNDATION BRUSH** blends to a flawless, full coverage look.

6. **SMALL STIFF CONCEALER BRUSH** maneuvers around your eye best.

7. **DOME BRONZER/BLUSH BRUSH** has long soft bristles that allow you to glide over foundation.

8. **ANGLED CONTOUR BRUSH** creates definition and hollow out cheeks.

9. **ROUND, SOFT POWDER BRUSH** for dusting powder on the face.

10. **ROUND, FLAT LIP BRUSH** creates a defined lip.

How to Clean Your Makeup Brushes like a Pro

Caring for your tools is an important part of creating a flawless beauty look. Ever try applying foundation with a brush that has makeup caked on it for weeks or months? Gross! Used an eyeliner brush that still has eyeliner from last night? It's pretty hard to maneuver. It's difficult to get a seamless look with dirty brushes—not to mention what you could get by using them, like acne or staph! No thanks. Besides, brushes are expensive. If you have purchased quality brushes, you will want to properly care for them to protect your investment. Clean your brushes once every one to two weeks depending on use.

You will need some shampoo/cleanser, water, and a towel.

1. Place a little soap in the palm of your hand and swirl the brush in it, then add warm water to create lather and clean the brush. Avoid getting the barrel of the brush wet as much as possible so it doesn't loosen the glue and lose bristles. Rinse the brush until the water runs clean. I use Dr. Bronner's 18-in-1 Hemp Lavender Pure-Castile Soap (EWG score: 0).

2. Gently squeeze the excess water out of the brush, keeping its original shape, then place it on a towel.

3. Once all the brushes are clean, use the towel to pat them dry.

4. Next, lay them flat along the edge of a counter so that the bristles hang over a bit and the air can circulate all the way around them.

5. Between washings you can spritz your brushes with a brush cleaner or hand sanitizer, such as Mineral Fusion Brush Cleaner (EWG score: 1)

+ **Pro Tip:** *Foundation, concealer, and lip brushes take a bit more product to clean them. Break down the product on the brushes a few minutes in advance with brush cleaner or oil, such as coconut oil. Let it sit while you clean your powder brushes first.*

+ **Pro Tip:** *To save time, group powder brushes together, like eye shadow and blush brushes. They are easy to clean and don't require a lot of extra product or washing.*

SKIN CARE

Mist/Toner

TAMMY FENDER BULGARIAN ROSE WATER (EWG score: 0*): Gently hydrates skin and has an intoxicating smell of roses.

URSA MAJOR 4-IN-1 ESSENTIAL FACE TONIC (EWG score: 2*): A refreshing, multitasking toner packed with nourishing botanicals that balance, exfoliate, hydrate, and repair your skin.

MARIE VERONIQUE MIST (EWG score: 1): Geared toward antiaging with DMAE, green tea, brightening, and anti-inflammatory ingredients.

Hydrators

ACURE ORGANICS ARGAN NIGHT CREAM (EWG score: 1): A lightweight night cream that is great for the summer months and for oily skin.

BEAUTYCOUNTER EVERYDAY AM HYDRATING CREAM (EWG score: 2): A lightweight moisturizer that absorbs quickly and doesn't feel tacky.

TAMMY FENDER INTENSIVE REPAIR BALM (EWG score: 3*, with two unknown ingredients): A cult classic for its intense repairing qualities. I use this on oversensitive skin.

Cleansers

BEAUTYCOUNTER NOURISHING CLEANSING BALM (EWG score: 2): A true balm that wipes away dirt and makeup, leaving your face hydrated enough you can skip the moisturizer. Comes with a handy cloth that exfoliates nicely.

MARIE VERONIQUE EXFOLIATING CLEANSER (EWG score: 2): A gentle exfoliating wash that is effective without disrupting the natural balance of your skin. Smells heavenly.

URSA MAJOR FANTASTIC FACE WASH (EWG score: 2*): A gentle exfoliator that cleans without drying. Has an earthy cedar smell that I love.

AEOS CLEANSING OIL (EWG score: 0*): Superdelicate on the skin but thorough enough to take off makeup. Leaves your skin feeling silky.

LUMINANCE DELICATE CLEANSER (EWG score: 0): I like this because it is less greasy than an oil but not a harsh as some foaming cleansers. Two mists does the trick.

Oils

TATA HARPER BEAUTIFYING FACE OIL (EWG score: 2): Brown algae revives fatigued skin. Dries down dewy but not greasy.

SKIN OWL BEAUTY DROPS (EWG score: 0*): Antibacterial and anti-inflammatory properties makes this a great choice for blemished skin.

SUNDAY RILEY JUNO HYDROACTIVE CELLULAR FACE OIL (EWG score: 0*): Fights aging with natural retinol, omega and amino acids, and vitamin C for luminous skin.

KARI GRAN ESSENTIAL SERUM (EWG score: 1): Nourishing botanicals and vitamin E hydrate the skin for a radiant glow.

Antiaging

ACURE RADICAL WRINKLE COMPLEX (EWG score: 1*): A generous amount of Chlorella Growth Factor (CGF) helps cell renewal, and you can say bye-bye to dull skin.

DERMA *e* DEEP WRINKLE PEPTIDE SERUM (EWG score: 2): Skip the Botox—this sophisticated serum helps muscles relax and smooths deep wrinkles.

MAD HIPPIE VITAMIN C SERUM (EWG score: 1): An amazing C serum that helps tone skin and fade dark spots. Plus, it has hyaluronic acid to plump the skin—it's so good.

ODACITÉ PA + G HYPERPIGMENTATION (EWG score: 0): Papaya enzymes combined with geranium and lemon works fast to fade hyperpigmentation and even out skin tone.

LARÉNIM DUSK TIL DAWN RECOVERY (EWG score: 0): Niacinamide aids flushed, blemished, and aging skin to restore a healthy radiance.

RESTORSEA REPAIRING NECK AND DÉCOLLETAGE CREAM (EWG score: 2*): If you need a serum to make your chest look more like your youthful, pampered face, this is the one.

EYES

Eye Gel/Serum

OSEA EYE GEL SERUM (EWG score: 2): An antioxidant-rich formula that tightens, firms, and reduces puffiness with marine-based extracts and resveratrol.

ANDALOU NATURALS LUMINOUS EYE SERUM BRIGHTENING (EWG score: 1): A light gel that utilizes fruit stem cells and green coffee to flush out water retention and reduce dark circles.

EMERGINC SCIENTIFIC ORGANICS EYELIGHT SERUM (EWG score: 1): Roll-on eye serum that nourishes, brightens, and hydrates with superantioxidants and grape stem cells.

DR. HAUSCHKA EYE REVIVE (EWG score: 1): Formulated with eyebright to relieve tired, red, puffy eyes. Excellent for dry eyes.

Eye Cream

WELEDA WILD ROSE SOOTHING EYE CREAM (EWG score: 1): A lightweight cream with a delicate rose fragrance. Good for sensitive eyes.

EVAN HEALY CHAMOMILE EYE CARE CREAM (EWG score: 1): Absorbs fast and provides generous hydration and decreased puffiness.

ODACITE ODACITÉ ULTRA EFFECTIVE EYE CREAM (EWG score: 1): Hyaluronic acid, vitamin E, and plum soften fine lines.

ECCO BELLA NATURAL EYE NUTRIENTS CREAM (EWG score: 2): Just a few drops of this lutein, lycopene, astaxanthin, CoQ10, vitamins E and C–rich cream refreshes tired eyes.

SCRUBS/EXFOLIATORS

Manual

TAMMY FENDER EXFOLIATOR EPI PEEL (EWG score: 2*): A fabulous skin polisher. The fine scrub buffs and brightens to perfection with a soft, hydrated finish.

DERMA *e* MICRODERMABRASION SCRUB (EWG score: 2): You will be surprised that this gentle scrub exfoliates every bit as well as the machine with amazing results.

S.W. BASICS EXFOLIANT (EWG score: 0*): Fine grains of oat, almond, and sea salt slough away dead skin cells, leaving you with smooth, glowing skin.

Chemical

ANDALOU NATURALS KOMBUCHA ENZYME EXFOLIATING PEEL (EWG score: 1): Kombucha enzymes exfoliate and soften, yet it's gentle enough for most skin types.

ARCONA CRANBERRY GOMMAGE EXFOLIATE AM (EWG score: 1): Cranberry and raspberry enzymes loosen dead skin cells while fine grit brilliantly sloughs off dry, flaky skin.

JUICE BEAUTY APPLE PEEL (EWG score: 2): A celebrity favorite and for good reason—this peel exfoliates! I can feel it working and sometimes get gentle flaking.

Masks

MAY LINDSTROM SKIN PROBLEM SOLVER (EWG score: 0*): This spicy concoction is one of my favorites. It tightens pores, reduces inflammation, and increases circulation.

DR. ALKAITIS ORGANIC UNIVERSAL MASK (EWG score: 1,* with ten unknown botanicals): I love all Dr. Alkaitis products, but they are impossible to score due to so many mysterious botanicals, such as Magical Forest Mushroom Complex (consisting of Snow,* Tuckahoe,* Hedgehog,* and Immortality* mushrooms). Still, I trust them and am quite amused.

DR. HAUSCHKA CLARIFYING CLAY MASK (EWG score: 0): I love this old school–style clay mask that purifies and draws out toxins.

NATUROPATHICA ALOE REPLENISHING GEL MASK (EWG score: 1*): A soothing anti-inflammatory mask that hydrates and plumps with hyaluronic acid.

PRATIMA NEEM SOOTHING MASK (EWG score: 0): A potent ayurvedic blend to heal blemishes, absorb excess oil, and calm the skin.

Acne

EVAN HEALY BLEMISH TREATMENT SERUM (EWG score: 0): A speedy and effective blemish treatment.

MYCHELLE DERMACEUTICALS WHITE CRANBERRY CLEANSER ACNE/OILY SKIN (EWG score: 2): Cleanses with drying, like many acne washes. Has a gorgeous citrus smell.

ALBA BOTANICA ACNEDOTE DEEP PORE WASH (EWG score: 2): An excellent scrub/wash combo that exfoliates with salicylic acid and controls oil.

ODACITÉ OILY ACNE PRONE BOOSTER (EWG score: 0): A deep, penetrating, purifying booster that would complement any blemish-prone skin care routine.

LIP BALM

S.W. BASICS ORGANIC LIP BALM PEPPERMINT (EWG score: 0*):
Highly emollient and hydrating without being too greasy. I love
the cool peppermint feel.

KARI GRAN LIP WHIP (EWG score: 1): Deeply moisturizing and
makes a great base for your preferred lip treatment.

ECO LIPS SOFTENING LIP BALM RELIEVE, COCOA VANILLA NUT
(EWG score: 0*): A wonderfully hydrating lip balm that is satiny smooth and smells like Grandma's house.

MAKEUP REMOVER

S.W. BASICS MAKEUP REMOVER (EWG score: 0): An olive oil
based remover that leaves your skin soft and moisturized. Works
well on eye makeup too.

MINERAL FUSION EYE MAKEUP REMOVER (EWG score: 2): A gel
formula that works as well as an oil for taking off tough eye
makeup.

**PHYSICIANS FORMULA ORGANIC WEAR EYE MAKEUP REMOVER
LIQUID** (EWG score: 1): Smells lightly of lavender and works
like a charm on stubborn eye makeup without the greasy residue.

LIVING NATURE GENTLE MAKEUP REMOVER (EWG score: 0):
Great for sensitive skin by gently removing makeup and grim.
This is not an eye makeup remover.

HAIR CARE

Styling Products

RAHUA VOLUMINOUS HAIR SPRAY (EWG score: 2): This is not your momma's hairspray. It gives a light hold and feels soft, not crisp. Great for adding texture and as a root lifter.

YAROK FEED YOUR ROOTS MOUSSE (EWG score: 3*): Adds volume to limp, lifeless hair while adding vitamins and nutrients to your scalp and hair.

JOHN MASTERS ORGANICS SEA MIST SEA SALT SPRAY WITH LAVENDER (EWG score: 0): This is great to add texture to wash-and-go styles or before your blowout.

ACURE ORGANICS DRY SHAMPOO (EWG score: 0*): I love the component. It delivers fine puffs of powder with no mess. A few dustings at the root peps up my tired, oily hair.

Shampoo

RARE EL'EMENTS PURE SHAMPOO (EWG score: 1): I always get compliments on how great my hair smells when I use this scalp treatment, shampoo, and conditioner.

HUGO NATURALS SMOOTHING AND DEFINING COCONUT SHAMPOO (EWG score: 1): Cleanses thoroughly without suds and a light coconut scent, leaving hair silky and smooth.

SHEA MOISTURE ORGANIC RAW SHEA BUTTER MOISTURE RETENTION SHAMPOO (EWG score: 1): Argan and shea butter help restore overprocessed and damaged hair, leaving it soft and manageable.

INTELLIGENT NUTRIENTS HARMONIC SHAMPOO (EWG score: 2): A gentle and lathering shampoo that smells amazing and can double as a body wash.

Conditioner

RARE EL'EMENTS ESSENTIAL LITE CONDITIONER DAILY MASK (EWG score: 1*): Leaves my thick, wavy hair shiny and silky.

JOHN MASTERS ORGANICS HONEY & HIBISCUS HAIR RECON-STRUCTOR (EWG score: 2): Hydrates and smooths ends. Good for color-treated hair.

AUBREY ORGANICS CHAMOMILE LUXURIOUS VOLUMIZING CON-DITIONER (EWG score: 2): Leaves even the finest hair shiny, smooth, and detangled without weighing it down.

Masks/Oils/Treatments

HAMADI ORGANICS SHEA HAIR CREAM (EWG score: 2*): Leaves your hair soft, shiny, and manageable. A little goes a long way with this cream.

LA BELLA FIGURA BOHEMIA VERDE AROMATIC HAIR (EWG score: 1*): I like to use just a dab of this to tame flyaways.

ACURE ORGANICS MOISTURIZING ROOT REPAIR DEEP CONDITION-ING HAIR MASK (EWG score: 1): Conditions without weighing hair down and is mild enough to use daily. Smells minty clean.

RAHUA FINISHING TREATMENT (EWG score: 2): Repairs and protects damaged hair and leaves a pretty gloss that's not greasy or heavy if used correctly.

ISUN SOOTHING HERBAL HAIR OIL (EWG score: 1*): Argan oil and ayurvedic herbs calm and sooth scalp. A wonderful choice for those with scalp problems.

NAIL CARE

5-Free Nail Polish

DEBORAH LIPPMANN: Fashion's darling for a good reason. Super-sophisticated colors and high shine make these lacquers standouts.

JENNA HIPP: A color collection from one of the hippest nail artists in Hollywood. Her 12 mini nail lacquers are a must have for every girl. I love Tweet Me!

RGB: Pretty chip resistant colors from fashionable partnerships from cool artists such as Jennifer Fisher.

SHESWAI: A lovely boutique line of high-quality lacquers in gorgeous colors. The bottles are so pretty!

SCOTCH NATURALS: They coined the phrase "all free" with their NaturaLaq, The only nature-based nail lacquer. A water-based polish that performs like a traditional one.

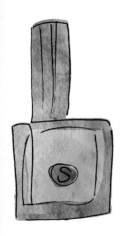

ZOYA: What I love about this company is that they are so fun. They are always on-trend.

PRITI NYC: Another clever boutique line of cool colors. The Princess collection is awesome for kids—they glow in the dark!

ELLA + MILA: I love the mommy-and-me sets. The company's motto is "polish with love." Cute!

Remover/Treatment

PRITI NYC SOY NAIL POLISH REMOVER (EWG score: 1*): A wonderful alternative to traditional polish removers. Effectively removes polish without harsh chemicals.

SCOTCH NATURALS NON-TOXIC NAIL POLISH REMOVER (EWG score: 1*): Made for their water-based polishes but can be used on others if you don't mind working a bit harder.

DEBORAH LIPPMANN INTENSIVE NAIL TREATMENT (EWG score: 1): Not only strengthens nails but acts as a nice base coat for polish.

RGB NAIL CARE IN CUTICLE OIL (EWG score: 0): Nourishes chapped, cracked skin and dry cuticles.

SPARITUAL CUTI-CLEAN CUTICLE AND STAIN REMOVER (EWG score: 1): Softens and removes dead skin and those pesky stains.

BATH & BODY

Scrubs

S.W. BASICS BODY SCRUB (EWG score: 0*): Gentle, softening, and smells so good (with only three ingredients), you'll want to eat it.

DEEP STEEP ORGANIC SUGAR SCRUB PASSION FRUIT GUAVA (EWG score: 2): It has a nice, creamy texture so it leaves your skin supersoft and moisturized.

NOURISH ORGANIC BODY POLISH (EWG score: 1): A USDA Organic polish that's a gentler exfoliant than salt or sugar scrub and loaded with nourishing ingredients.

Body Oils

DR. HAUSCHKA ROSE NURTURING BODY OIL (EWG score: 0): One of my favorites for its beautiful, not overpowering rose scent.

INDIE LEE PATCHOULI SANDALWOOD MOISTURIZING OIL (EWG score: 0): A wonderful nongreasy body oil that I have also used to tame any frizz in my hair.

TATA HARPER REVITALIZING BODY OIL (EWG score: 1): I love that I can get dressed immediately after using this oil.

Lotions

SHEA MOISTURE RAW SHEA BUTTER LOTION (EWG score: 2): This soothed my chapped skin beautifully, and a little goes a long way.

EVAN HEALY WHIPPED SHEA BUTTER WITH OLIVE LEAF (EWG score: 1): This butter has a light and creamy texture that soaks right in.

S.W. BASICS CREAM (EWG score: 0): A rich shea butter–based cream that deeply penetrates to soften dry skin.

ALBA BOTANICA VERY EMOLLIENT BODY LOTION (EWG score: 3): Very hydrating and not greasy.

Shower Gels

SHEAMOISTURE COCONUT & HIBISCUS FOAMING MILK & BODY WASH (EWG score: 2): This wash is highly moisturizing and gentle enough to use on my baby too.

LIVING NATURE NOURISHING BODY WASH (EWG score: 1): A very gentle gel that contains manuka honey that has fantastic antiseptic properties.

ANDALOU NATURALS CLEMENTINE GINGER ENERGIZING SHOWER GEL (EWG score: 2): A nice, mild wash with a very subtle fragrance.

BURTS BEES FABULOUSLY FRESH BODY WASH (EWG score: 3): Energizing and refreshing, a great way to start the day.

Soaps

PANGEA ORGANICS BAR SOAP ITALIAN WHITE SAGE, GERANIUM & YARROW (EWG score: 1): Has a wonderfully fresh, clean scent and is highly moisturizing.

OUT OF AFRICA PURE SHEA BUTTER BAR SOAP (EWG score: 0): Superbly moisturizing with a nice, rich lather.

DR. BRONNER'S 18 IN 1 HEMP LAVENDER PURE-CASTILE SOAP (EWG score: 0): A fantastic multiuse soap. I use this for many household cleaning needs.

Bath Soaks/Salt/Oil

AHAVA EUCALYPTUS BATH SALT (EWG score: 2): Transform your bath into a spa experience with this soak.

FIG + YARROW FLORAL MILK BATH SOAK (EWG score: 2*): Aromatic and ultramoisturizing with gentle exfoliation.

PRATIMA ROSE ORGANIC BATH OIL (EWG score: 0*): Improve your heart energy and promote love with rose oil while you hydrate and soften your skin.

SUN CARE

Sunscreen

GOLDFADEN MD SUN VISOR ULTRALIGHT OIL FREE SPF 30 MIST (EWG score: 3*): This works under or over makeup. Creates an unexpectedly pretty matte finish.

DIVITA NATURAL SKIN CARE SOLAR BODY BLOCK 30 SPF (EWG score: 1): I love the way this feels on my skin. It's a hydrator with all the benefits of a sunscreen and provides a 30 SPF.

VIVE SANA SOLAR TO POLAR (EWG score: 2): A sunscreen that acts like a BB cream. Works well alone or under makeup; superhydrating.

AUBREY ORGANICS PURE ALOE VERA (EWG score: 1): An ultra-soothing gel for face and body.

Bronzers/Self-Tanners

PRTTY PEAUSHUN SKIN TIGHT BODY LOTION DEEP DARK (EWG score: 3*): I love the subtle sheen this gives your skin. I use it on all my photo shoots.

TRUE NATURAL ANTI-AGING PERFECT TAN SELF-TAN LOTION (EWG score: 2*): What I first noticed about this is that it smells good and feels moisturizing. The color is pretty and natural looking.

CHOCOLATE SUN COCOA GLOW FACE AND BODY CREAM (EWG score 1*; with three unknown ingredients): This self-tanner is so good. It smells delicious and gives you the most gorgeous tan. People will think you've been on holiday.

LAVERA SELF-TANNING LOTION (EWG score: 3*): Gives my medium-toned skin a boost of color without looking orangey.

CHOCOLATE SUN COCOA ILLUME FACE GEL (EWG score: 1*): If you want a natural-looking tan on your face, this gel nails it.

HAIR REMOVAL

MOOM NATURAL WAX STRIPS (EWG score: 0): Easy to use, works great, and as a bonus, each strip can be used more than once.

PARISSA PERSIAN COLD WAX (EWG score: 0): Removes coarse hair and works well when it's warmed too.

SHEA MOISTURE WAX HONEY SUGAR (EWG score: 3): Natural anti-inflammatories minimizes ingrown hairs and skin irritation. Water-soluble wax makes cleanup easy.

The Vault

I am opening the vault for you here and sharing some über luxurious green beauty products. To come up with this list of premium products, I enlisted the help of my friend Stacey Stilts, founder of Green Line Beauty in Los Angeles.

SAMADARA ULTIMATE AGE-DEFYING CRÈME (EWG score: 0*): A potent antiaging treatment that incorporates two rose quartz crystals.

SODASHI VANILLA BODY BUTTER (EWG score: 0*): A luxurious moisturizing butter that smells divinely of its namesake vanilla.

RESTORSEA 24KT LIQUID GOLD FACE OIL (EWG score: 2*): With real gold flakes this oil gives you a gorgeous glow while hydrating and controlling oil production.

TAMMY FENDER QUINTESSENTIAL SERUM (EWG score: 1*): Touted as an "all-in-one age-defying superstar."

TATA HARPER IRIDESCENT REVITALIZING BODY OIL (EWG score: 2*): Imparts your skin with a subtle bronze sheen.

RODIN OLIO LUSSO LUXURY FACE OIL (EWG score: 2*): A fragrant lightweight oil with a cult following. Absorbs quickly and softens skin.

Gorgeously Green Beauty Boxes

PETIT VOUR delivers fresh beauty miniatures culled from beauty's kindest. Earn points with purchases, reviews and friend recommendations.

GOODEBOX a discovery box that provides healthy beauty products, nontoxic and natural cosmetics and personal care products.

SPA HEROES delivers spa-sourced discoveries for skin, hair, and body made with good-for-you ingredients.

Natural/Organic Fragrance

PACIFICA These are fun, fresh, and totally affodable.

STRANGE INVISIBLE Intoxicating perfumes that keep you wanting to try more.

AURA-SAMA A liquid elixir that's pure joy. My favorite is No. 39.

LURK These fragrances smell devine and are unisex.

INTELLIGENT NUTRIENTS Heavenly and clever perfumes. Certified organic smart armor perfume spray is genius.

HONORÉ DES PRÉS Ubür chic French perfumes—they do perfume so well.

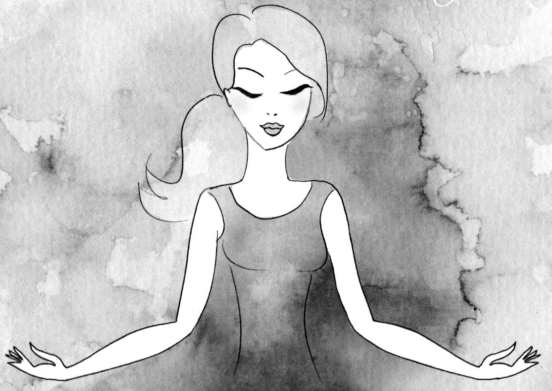

Chapter Eight

Paige's
TOP TEN Beauty
Secrets

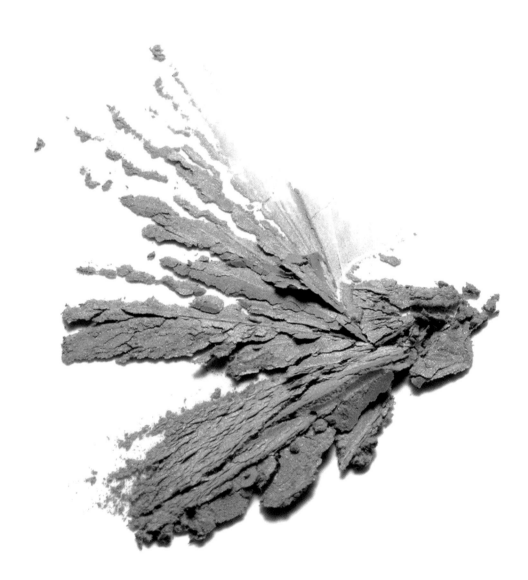

I said early on in the book that I believe beauty comes from confidence. That is my universal beauty philosophy, which transcends whatever products you use. I believe every woman is beautiful. Confidence doesn't always come easily, but there are some basic things every woman can do to feel confident and look her best. It goes without saying that you should get enough sleep, stay well hydrated, eat a balanced diet of whole foods, exercise regularly, don't smoke, and enjoy your vices in moderation. These acts are essential to looking good and feeling your best. In addition to this foundation to vibrant health and beauty, there are small changes in your beauty routine you can make to help you feel confident and look gorgeous. Here are my top ten go-to beauty secrets to keep you glowing.

GREEN BEAUTY SECRET NO. 1: PAMPER YOUR SKIN

There is nothing more gorgeous (or healthy looking) than radiant skin. The elements, environment, hormones, stress, skin disorders, and your diet all contribute to the health and appearance of your complexion. Your skin changes over the decades as you age. The concerns you have when you are in your teens won't be the same as when you are in your thirties. Many of these issues are universal, like antiaging and dry skin. There are some basic things you can do to help your skin look and feel its best for decades to come.

Teens

All teenagers know what acne is. So many girls try to dry it out and cover it with heavy makeup, but that's not the best approach. Rather than drying out your skin and looking parched, give it some hydration. Besides, the more you dry out your skin, the more oil it will produce. Your skin needs to be hydrated. Look for oil-free moisturizers and stick to mineral-based sunscreens. Go light on the makeup whenever possible to let your skin breathe. If you must cover acne, make sure you prep your skin so it's well hydrated and primed. You will use less foundation and your makeup will look prettier.

> **INCORPORATE:** Cleanser, toner, moisturizer, broad spectrum SPF (sunscreen)

> **INGREDIENTS:** Zinc oxide, oil-free formulas, benzoyl peroxide

Twenties

The years from twenty to twenty-nine are great! Our skin is probably at its healthiest naturally, but wind, sun, and the changes between indoor and outdoor environments can cause a combination of problems. Certain parts of our face may seem oily, while others are dry and flaky. Our skin is maturing, and we need to adjust our skin care routine along with these changes. This is the time when you want to start practicing good skin care habits if you haven't been taking great care of your skin already. You want to preserve your youthful skin as long as possible. One of the best ways to do this is to wear sunscreen. The sun is wonderful and healthy in small doses, but too much exposure over time can wreak havoc on your youthful glow. You won't see the sun damage immediately, but trust me, you will in your thirties and forties.

Your skin may become more combination than oily or even dry in areas. At this point moisturizer is essential. If you still have acne, you may need to adjust your acne treatments to something less harsh. The acne you have in your twenties will be different than in your teens. It will likely be more on the jawline and hormonally based. No matter what your skin type is, in your twenties you should avoid harsh and drying products. Seek out products for combination skin and incorporate a moisturizer and sunscreen. During your twenties is also a good time to start using an eye cream to stave off crow's feet.

INCORPORATE: Moisturizer, eye cream

INGREDIENTS: Green tea extract, acai extract, and peptides

Thirties

If you have been diligent in your twenties with your skin care routine, your skin may not show major signs of aging. However, wrinkles begin to appear in our thirties—even if we can't quite see them yet. Our faces can start to look dull, and cell turnover is much slower. We start to see a loss of elasticity and collagen. The skin beneath our eyes may get darker or retain fluid. The sun damage from our teens and twenties becomes more prominent. For many of us, hyperpigmentation will become a top priority.

This is the time to get more aggressive with antiaging products. You don't have to use harsh chemicals like hydroquinone and retinol, but you may want to include a vitamin C serum in your skin care routine and perhaps more powerful antioxidants like resveratrol. It's also when you should be manually exfoliating with a gentle scrub or brush to encourage cell renewal. If you choose to use a retinol this is the decade to start. And don't forget your lips! Oil serums are great to help you keep a luminous glow. Keep doing all the good skin care in your thirties and stay on top of your broad spectrum SPF.

INCORPORATE: Antioxidant serum, manual exfoliator, eye
treatment/gel

INGREDIENTS: Vitamin A, C & E, resveratrol, CoQ10, caffeine,
hyaluronic acid, and oils like argan, jojoba, and passion fruit

Forties

Women with medium-dark to dark skin tones are now starting to
see the obvious signs of aging, such as lines, wrinkles, and collagen
loss. Light to medium-light skin tones are seeing more sun damage
than they did in their thirties. If you have been wearing sunscreen
regularly, this will be dramatically reduced than if you didn't. Skin
issues due to perimenopause arise at this time, such as sallowness,
dryness, and acne. Continue with all the antiaging ingredients from
your thirties, but toning, hydration, and nourishment are key. Keep
using your sunscreen, and don't forget your chest and the back of
your hands.

INCORPORATE: Cream cleanser, hydrating and toning serums

INGREDIENTS: Nourishing extracts such as grape seed, algae/sea-
weed, and evening primrose, which has gamma linolenic acid
(GLA) omega-6 fatty acid and niacinamide

Fifties-Plus

In this decade you will reap the benefits of taking such good care
of your skin and making healthy lifestyle choices. Your skin will be
at its driest and perhaps it will be flaky. You will notice thinner skin,
broken capillaries, and darker circles in the skin under your eyes. You
will have more color loss and sagging. Your lines and wrinkles have
deepened. It may sound frightening, but taking care of yourself will
minimize these signs of aging and keep you looking radiant no matter
what. Most important, your self-love and happiness will make you

look and feel beautiful. Hydration and softening are most important now. Continue with all the antioxidant serums and creams, but at this point in your life, hydration and softening become the focus.

INCORPORATE: Masks and night masks

INGREDIENTS: Oils from seeds, nuts, fruits and plants, rosehip seed oil, and apricot seed oil for softening

GREEN BEAUTY SECRET NO. 2: BE SAFE IN THE SUN

Wearing sunscreen is the best way to keep your skin gorgeous for years to come. Many people only use sunscreen when they are at the beach, lake, or poolside, but the American Cancer Society says that UV exposure adds up day after day every time you are in the sun, and getting too much sun can be harmful. They suggest wearing a daily broad-spectrum sunscreen of at least SPF 30, if you're going to be in direct sun for more than fifteen minutes. They also suggest seeking shade whenever possible and wearing proper clothing, including hats and sunglasses. Check! That's easy enough, but what if you want to get some sun? Do you know how to do that safely?

You should still wear sunscreen, a hat, and sunglasses, but the key to sunning safely is using a natural chemically safe sunscreen and knowing what to expect from your sunscreen. To get more or less UV rays, consider your SPF level. If you want more sun exposure and perhaps a little tan, consider a lower SPF. No matter what, always use a sunscreen if you are in direct sun for more than fifteen minutes, and reapply it every couple of hours and after you've been in the water, even if it says "waterproof" or "water resistant."

Sun Protection Factor (SPF) Scale:	
SPF 4	filters out 75 percent of UVB rays
SPF 10	filters out 90 percent of UVB rays
SPF 15	filters out 93 percent of UVB rays
SPF 30	filters out 97 percent of UVB rays
SPF 50	filters out 98 percent of UVB rays
SPF 100	filters out 99 percent of UVB rays

No sunscreen protects you completely. The higher the SPF factor, the smaller the difference becomes. There is not a huge difference between 30 and 50, so this is why it's not necessary to use higher than 30 SPF; it won't really make a difference. By understanding how sunscreens work, you will know how to use them to achieve the amount of sun you want.

The problem with sunscreens is that they can be overused, and the higher the SPF, the more toxic chemicals you expose yourself to. Additionally, SPF ingredients are endangering our marine life. This is another reason why you should wear protective clothing and use sunscreen only when and where you need it. A good pair of sunglasses should provide protection from 99 percent of UVB rays.

Now that you understand how to use sunscreen, let's learn how to find a chemically safe one. Here are some tips to help you find a safe and effective sunscreen. Watch out for:

• Chemical UV absorbers

• Titanium dioxide (spray on)

• Synthetic preservatives

- Oxybenzone

- Nanoparticles

- Retinyl palmitate (Vitamin A)

Seek out:

- Zinc oxide

- Natural preservatives

- Organic ingredients

- Broad spectrum that blocks UVB and UVA rays

One last note: never ever use tanning beds or booths. The International Agency for Research on Cancer shows that tanning is especially hazardous to young people. The use of sunbeds before the age of thirty increases your chance of melanoma by 75 percent.[12] It's not worth it!

Six Travel Must Haves

1. **SOAPWALLA ESSENTIAL FACIAL TONING MIST** (EWG score: 2*): A delicious rose geranium blend that smells and feels so refreshing.

2. **ANDALOU NATURALS FRUIT STEM CELL REVITALIZE SERUM** (EWG score: 1): This serum revives my skin and imparts a healthy glow.

3. **LULU ORGANICS LAVENDER + CLARY SAGE HAIR POWDER** (EWG score: 1*): I rub a little through my fingertips then run them through my roots for instantly fluffy hair.

4. **ACURE ORGANICS UNSCENTED ARGAN OIL CLEANSING TOW-ELETTES FOR FACE & BODY** (EWG score: 2*): Cleansing but gentle; perfect for a little pick-me-up or removing makeup.

5. **JOHN MASTERS LIP CALM** (EWG score: 1): One of my favorite lip balms for its amazing texture and hydration. I keep it by my bedside.

6. **THE HONEST COMPANY HAND SANITIZER SPRAY** (EWG score: 1): A superhandy spray that smells great—and it's quick-drying.

GREEN BEAUTY SECRET NO. 3: PREP AND PRIME

The key to flawless, glowing skin is skin preparation. Skin that is dry, oily, congested, puffy, and tired doesn't look healthy.

Prep

If you're following a good skin care regime, half your prep work is done. If not, you will need to clean, tone, and hydrate your face. If you have dry skin, you will need an intense hydrator. If it's oily, an oil-free moisturizer is best. For combination and normal skin, a lightweight or daytime hydrator should be fine. You can always add a heavier moisturizer in the areas that you need it.

Don't skip the toner; it will help you balance your skin's pH level and absorb the moisturizer. Remember: one way for skin to absorb a substance is to make sure it's well hydrated, so mist a toner, or at the very least water, on your face before you apply your moisturizer. When you apply your toner and hydrator, don't forget the ears, neck, and chest. If you have really oily skin, use a mattifier to control oil production throughout the day.

Your lips should be exfoliated and well hydrated before you apply any lip color. Use a lip balm to hydrate the lips and the area around and inside your nostrils by using a cotton swab and the balm. It is an area that is often neglected.

Prime

Primers are wonderful for creating a smooth matte, velvety, or dewy canvas. They can help you create any finish you desire. A primer provides a smooth canvas that allows the makeup to glide on, wear for hours longer, and stay where you put it. It creates a barrier to the skin so your skin doesn't absorb the makeup as quickly. It can also keep oil at bay. You don't always have to wear a primer, but I find that if I am wearing more than a little mascara and lip balm and want to apply a real beauty look, primers help the makeup application tremendously. Everything goes on better, and you have to use so much less because your skin already looks flawless. Find the right primer for your skin type by considering your specific needs. If your skin is dry, oily, or mature, choose a primer that is specifically formulated for those particular needs. Other primers are made to fight redness, minimize the appearance of pores, or reflect light.

Eye shadow primers work well, too. They will keep your eye shadow from creasing or disappearing throughout the day. They make your eye shadow brighter and they apply and blend more easily. Lip primers will extend the life of your lipstick application. They help create a smooth surface and enhance color. Lash primers work well for fragile or short lashes. Some condition while others lengthen. In general, primers give you a flawless finish with staying power.

Problem Solvers

PROBLEM: Sallow skin

SOLUTION: Use an oxygen treatment or mask that aids microcirculation, then apply an energizing or brightening serum followed by a hydrator.

PROBLEM: Not plump

SOLUTION: Apply a serum with hyaluronic acid followed by moisturizer.

PROBLEM: Not supple

SOLUTION: Use an intense hydration (water) gel mask followed by an oil serum/moisturizer.

PROBLEM: Dry skin or patches

SOLUTION: Apply a rich moisturizing mask twenty minutes before you start your makeup.

PROBLEM: Puffy eyes

SOLUTION: Apply an eye gel twenty minutes before you start your makeup.

PROBLEM: Dark circles

SOLUTION: Apply an eye cream with vitamin K that promotes microcirculation. Use a correcting concealer.

PROBLEM: Tired

SOLUTION: Rub an ice cube over your face after you apply your makeup just before you leave the house. Bring light to your eyes with brightening pens or pencils.

GREEN BEAUTY SECRET NO. 4: BRIGHTEN UP!

C onsider concealer your secret weapon. It can instantly take years off your face. It can help you look rested even if you've been up all night with your newborn baby, pulled an all-nighter for the boss, or celebrated till dawn with friends. With one swipe of a brush, your blue veins, ruptured capillaries, and brown spots can be gone. If you have concealer in your cosmetic bag, you will never gasp over dark under-eye circles or a blemish again. All you have to do is conceal and brighten in all the right places.

Color

Different colors do different things. Yellow neutralizes blue, green cancels out red, and so on. Most people, myself included, aren't going to take the time to use the various colors to correct (neutralize color) first. I prefer to use a concealer that acts like a corrector. To correct the dark under-eye area, use a concealer color that has peach or pink undertones depending on your skin tone. It should also closely match your skin tone or the tone of your foundation if you are using one. One shade lighter is fine, but if it's too light or too yellow, it could make you look ashy or give you raccoon eyes. Yellow and toned concealer works best for bringing light to the center of the face, highlighting, and covering blemishes.

Your skin is not the same color all year long. It's best to have two different colors to match your face in the winter and summer. You will need to blend the two between seasons to deepen or lighten your changing skin color.

Consistency

To cover under-eye circles, a creamy hydrating formula with a slight dewy finish works best for the delicate skin around the eye. You won't have to drag your skin to apply it, and it won't look dry and cakey. If you're looking to brighten your eyes, use a sheerer liquid formula with light-reflecting particles that will brighten and illuminate your face. If you are covering a blemish, use a drier pigment-rich formula to neutralize any redness. Stick formulas work well for this as long as they are opaque.

✦ **Pro Tip:** *When covering under-eye circles, prep with an eye cream first so your skin is as hydrated as possible. Allow it to soak in a few minutes, then neutralize the color under your eye using a concealer brush or your finger, starting at the inner corner. Use the least amount possible to achieve the look. Use downward strokes and blend well. Avoid using horizontal or crescent-shaped strokes. You can always build it if you need more coverage.*

✦ **Pro Tip:** *To conceal blemishes, use two colors and dot them directly on top of the blemish with a small pointed brush to camouflage it. Brush out the edges to blend the concealer. Set it and take down shine with a light layer of fine, translucent setting powder.*

Fake a Good Night's Sleep

Have you been partying like a rock star or moonlighting and burning the candle at both ends? If so, you are in good company. We have all been there. Consider me your partner in crime and follow these easy tips to fake having a restful night's sleep. And when you can, try to get some serious shuteye.

1. **DEPUFF:** Smear on a good under-eye gel or eye cream formu-
    lated to depuff your eyes. I like Derma *e* Soothing Eye Gel
    (EWG score: 2). It depuffs, plumps fine lines, and soothes the
    delicate under-eye area.

2. **HYDRATE—INSIDE AND OUT.** It's obvious but it's easy to for-
    get. Drink lots of water and keep your skin looking fresh with
    moisturizer. Dewey skin can take off years. Try Luminance
    Deep Hydration Facial Moisturizer (EWG score: 0*). Together,
    tamarind seed and tamanu oils act very much like collagen and
    gives skin a youthful, supple appearance. Yes, please!

3. **CONCEAL.** Hide unsightly dark circles with an under-eye
    concealer. If it's not specifically for the eyes, it could be too dry.
    You want a satin texture that has enough coverage but is not
    too matte. Tarte Maracuja Creaseless Concealer (EWG score:
    2) gives flawless skin. It has the perfect blend of coverage and
    hydration. Unlike many concealers that can be drying or heavy,
    this formula enhances and nourishes the skin.

4. **ILLUMINATE.** Bring light to your face with illuminators and
    highlighters. They come in cream, powder, liquid, and mousse
    form and are a girl's best friend. It's like an instant face-lift! You
    can use them on the eyes, cheeks, lips, and nose to add a fresh
    sheen. Use Jane Iredale Eye Highlighter Pencil (EWG score: 1)
    to add a soft glow to your face.

5. **BRIGHTEN.** Add a little color to your face with a bright lipstick
    or blush. A rose or coral color will warm up the skin and make
    you look alive and radiant. Revolution Organics Freedom Glow
    Beauty Balm, Sunkissed (EWG score: 1) gives the perfect flush
    every time! Love it!

GREEN BEAUTY SECRET NO. 5: LIGHTEN UP!

Less is more when it comes to makeup. It should never look like a mask. Makeup should enhance your features, not overpower them. Sure, it's a great way to cheat your imperfections, but you want people to notice *you* first and not your makeup.

- Conceal simply. Spot treating on a day-to-day basis is the best way to get a natural look.

- If you want a little coverage, opt for a tinted moisturizer or BB cream. I rarely use foundation on myself. I use a tinted moisturizer or BB cream on my face that's usually a touch darker than my skin tone to warm up my skin. This is trickier to do with foundation.

- If you want more or full coverage, use foundation sparingly and blend well. Foundation should disappear into your skin. You should never be able to see it on your face. It should blend seamlessly into your skin. Your face should match your neck. To find your shade color, stripe three colors on your jawline. The one that disappears into your skin tone is the correct one for you.

- Use a primer that works well for you and you will be able to use less foundation.

- Go easy on the powder and powder foundation. A matte finish is gorgeous, but cakey is unattractive.

- Make sure you have good lighting to apply your makeup. It will make a huge difference. When you walk outside, it should look good, not garish.

- If you get lipstick or lip gloss on your teeth, you have applied too much. Blot your lips on a paper towel after applying to avoid this.

- One eye shadow shade is plenty, but whatever you do, *never ever* use more than three colors.

- Avoid spidery eyelashes. If you want to wear false lashes, keep them natural looking. Use a mix of short and medium individual lashes for the most natural look. Strip lashes can be gorgeous and transform your look if done correctly, but often they ruin a beautiful look by looking too costumey.

GREEN BEAUTY SECRET NO. 6: GROOM YOUR BROWS

Eyebrows frame your face and have a huge impact on the way you look. They can make you look more youthful. A pretty arch can open your eye and give your face a lift. Poorly executed arches can make you look older or ghoulish, and sometimes downright scary. Eyebrow trends tend to be dramatic—either superthick or nothing at all. Neither tends to look great on most people. Rather than following the trends, focus on a brow that suits you best. I tell my clients to keep their brows on the fuller side. Fuller brows "read" more youthful. However, a full brow for you may not be the same as a full brow for your best friend or sister. Everyone's natural arch and thickness is different. I have seen women with brows that look great and natural on them but would look thin and too sparse on me. Bone structure has a lot to do with it, too. If you can find an amazing arch expert, you are golden. If not, maintain your own brows. Here's how.

Eyebrow Grooming Tools:

- Brow scissors

- Slant tweezers

- Brow pencil

- Spoolie brush

Eyebrow Grooming Instructions:

1. Mark your starting point to avoid overtweezing in the middle of your brows. The front (inside edge) of your brow should align with the top outside edge of your nose. Use your tweezers to find the line and a brow pencil to mark it.

2. An easy way not to overtweeze is to fill in the brow first then tweeze around the shape. Brush hairs up with a spoolie brush and fill in brows underneath. Hold your tweezers from the front of the brow to where the arch begins. If there is any space, fill that in with a brow pencil. Let it grow if possible. If it won't grow, don't stress—that's what brow pencils are made for.

3. Tweeze the stray hair around your shape. Never tweeze from the top of the brow unless you are an expert. It will ruin your natural arch and lower your eyebrows, which is the opposite of what you want to achieve.

4. The arch should begin just after the highest point of the brow. Where your natural brow peaks then tapers down is where you want to give a gentle arch. If you try to arch in the middle directly under the peak, you get joker eyebrows. It's more attractive and gives a prettier lift when you have a soft arch under your temples.

5. Once you have your shape, if you find you need a bit of a trim, using your spoolie brush, comb brows up and trim hairs that are longer than the others. Some variation is good; they don't need to be blunt. Snip only the tips where needed—don't overdo it.

6. Last, go for symmetry. They are sisters, not twins. If you have one eyebrow that is sparser than the other, don't overtweeze the fuller one to look like the other. It's fine if they are not identical, as long as they have symmetry.

GREEN BEAUTY SECRET NO. 7: DEVELOP A SIGNATURE LOOK

Celebrities have them and so can you! J.Lo has the glow. Gwen Stefani and Rita Ora rock red lips. Taylor Swift loves inky eyeliner. Zooey Deschanel wears doe-eyed long lashes. Kate Middleton sports rosy cheeks. Karlie Kloss and Halle Berry stand out in smoky eyes. Find a look that works for you. This should be your go-to look for when you need to look and feel your best. Once you have that as your core look, you can experiment.

Your signature look should be something you are comfortable with on a daily basis. It also tells a little about who you are and is a look you don't have to overthink, that you feel confident wearing, and best represents you. Your signature look will likely change over the years, and that's fine. The idea is to have a look that works for you now that you feel confident in. My signature look has changed over the years and changes with the season. However, I have always had a signature feature that I play up—my eyebrows. If you have a feature you love, embrace it. Display it. Showcase it. It makes you unique and alluring. Don't have a signature look? No worries. You can develop one.

How to Develop Your Signature Look:

1. Your makeup look will reflect who you are. Are you glamorous, romantic, sweet, girl next-door, preppy, earthy, sexy, classy, serious, all-American, effortlessly chic, or urban? You don't have to play this straight, but your signature look should give away something about you, a nuance about your personality. It sounds like a tall order, but it will naturally be there already—or you will simply draw it out.

2. If you have a feature you love, start there. Work your signature look around it. Wear fabulous glasses? Try a bold lip look. Have striking eye color? Wear a shadow that brightens them. Have amazing cheekbones? Wear a gorgeous contoured look. The options are endless. No doubt you have a few to try out. But you'll choose one for your signature look. How will you know?

3. Wear the different looks out in the world. Find out which look you like best. See how people respond to you and what your friends say. Ultimately, the one you feel most confident in is going to be the one that is right for you—your signature look.

GREEN BEAUTY SECRET NO. 8: BE BOLD

L ove to play with makeup but don't want to end up looking like the Joker? It's fun to try out different beauty looks. Like trying on new clothes, a new beauty look can take you from pretty to pretty fabulous. I love getting glammed up to go out to dinner, a concert, or a wedding. Whatever the occasion, for me it's a chance to reinvent myself with a new beauty look.

Now that you have a signature look, why not try something more adventurous. I love these four bold looks that never go out of style. They may not all be for you, but you should be able to wear one or two of them with confidence.

A Pop of Color on the Eyes

This is a fun way to incorporate a bold color and change up your look. However, done wrong, you could end up looking like a Harajuku Girl, which would be amazing, if that were the look you were going for. If not, here are some techniques to help you out.

1. **USE ONE COLOR.** Select a color that you love and that looks good on your skin and use only that color. If you don't cover your entire eye in the color, the rest should be bare.

2. **BE DELIBERATE.** Whether you want it on your top lid, lower lid, or both, strategic placement will make the look polished. The way you apply the color will make a difference in the way it is enhanced. If you want drama, go for a dark color.

3. **USE RESTRAINT.** If you want a pop of color on the eyelid, make sure it's expedited well. You don't have to apply color on the entire eye or all the way around for it to be pretty. Sometimes the best way to play with color is to strategically draw a blue wash of color on the lid without going past the crease.

4. **BALANCE A BRIGHT EYE WITH A NEUTRAL LIP.** That way the focus is only on the eyes.

A Bold Lip

Unless you are a pro, don't pair a bold lip with colorful eye shadow. It can be done, but it's hard to pull off unless you know exactly how to do it. Instead, stick to a neutral eye shadow in the brown or bronze tones, depending on the lip color. A stain is the easiest to apply when you are going bright red or superbold. You don't have to worry so much about a perfect line or getting it on right. You can use lipstick, too, to achieve the look by applying it straight from the tube then blotting your lips together to create a natural line and stain. Use a blotting paper to lift any emollients, leaving only pigment behind. To get maximum staying power, try using a tint first and then layer on a lipstick. Make sure the rest of your face is in balance with your bold lip by keeping it minimal.

Graphic Eyeliner

Heavily lined eyes are always in fashion. The cat eye is a classic look and has taken on many incarnations, but today's graphic liner is about color and beautiful lines (or dots). You don't have to sport liner like Amy Winehouse (but that would be amazing). A little extra liner strategically placed will do the trick. Next time you want to experiment, try these sweet styles.

- The white eyeliner trend looks so fresh. It's also easy to do and looks good on all ages. For the freshest look, simply line the top lash line—no need to wing it. It looks best kept on the lash line.

- If you want to go a bit bolder, try lining the lash line with a bright color or a metallic.

- For a more dramatic evening look, use a gel liner to draw a solid line across your top and bottom lash line. Then connect them with little triangles at the outer corner to create almond-shaped eyes.

- If you want to try something a bit more daring, draw a white (or any color) line on the lower lash line starting about halfway in to the outer corner and just beyond, then place a dot in the inner or outer corner for a cool element of surprise.

A Smoky Eye

Another beauty classic, the smoky eye is the go-to look for sexy, smoldering eyes. I will never forget the time I did my mother's makeup when I was working one of my first jobs at a glamour shots–type studio in Palm Springs. Those studios were all the rage in the 1990s! One day, as a surprise, I brought her into the studio, gave her a makeover, and took her pictures. She looked amazing, and her photos turned out beautifully . . . or so I thought. Because when she saw the photographs, she said I should have done more of a smoky eye. Hilarious! Mother always knows best.

To make the look more modern, try these techniques:

- Create a smoky bronze eye. Using bronze eye shadow, apply it on top of the lid just past the crease, wrapping it around to the bottom lash line. Blend well. Skip liner altogether for a minimal chic look.

- If you want to use liner, stick to a color that is monochromatic. Tone on tone looks fresh. A tone on tone mascara is also fun, but black works well with this look—just no black liner, please.

- Try this look with color. It also looks great in a deep saturated green, purple, or blue.

GREEN BEAUTY SECRET NO. 9: SMILE

Smiling is so important in daily life. Everyone is more beautiful when they smile. A smile is infectious. It has the ability to change the way others may perceive you. People are more drawn to those who smile big. I found this out firsthand in college. I went to a party where I didn't know anyone, and I felt so uncomfortable because I was really out of my element, not because I didn't know anyone (I make friends out of Uber drivers), but because they were of a much higher social class. I felt like a fish out of water. To hide that I was uncomfortable and give me an air of confidence, I smiled all night. Even when I was standing alone not talking to anyone, I was smiling. I was smiling at others and making eye contact. I kept telling myself, *Just smile*. And it worked. I really did feel more confident by smiling and saying a few silent mantras. Years later a woman from the party told me that all she could remember was me because I was smiling every time she looked at me and that I looked so pretty smiling. I will never forget that. It showed me how much power a smile had.

Some of us are blessed with a beautiful smile naturally. Others, like me, not so much. Don't get me wrong. It's not bad, but it is asymmetrical. I had to learn where my lips should fall, how to part my teeth, and to lift the side that was lazy. But smiling doesn't come easy for some people, including me. I don't mean we can't or don't want to smile, but knowing how to smile the way it looks best for you can be tricky. Seriously. It sounds so simple, but just like knowing your angles when taking a photo (apparently one side of my face takes ten pounds off me) you have to know what your best smile looks like. And I am not alone. It's been rumored that Mariah Carey will only be shot from one side. We all have our good side and we all have our best smile.

Do you know how to smile to best suit your face? If not, spend a little time in the mirror practicing. I have given you some things to consider when you are at the mirror. It won't matter so much on a day-to-day basis, but when you want to feel confident, look your best, or take photos, you'll be happy you spent the time thinking about it. While a smile in itself is beautiful, there is a lot you can do to smile your personal best.

- Practice your smile in front of the mirror. Look at your teeth. Pay attention to where they fall and how much they show. When you find your best smile, practice it until you can do it in your sleep. Do routine checkups, too. If it doesn't come naturally, you will forget it if you don't practice it with some regularity.

- Teeth matter. Brushing and flossing daily will keep them healthy and clean. If they are yellow or stained, try some over-the-counter whiteners. They will do wonders for your pearly whites.

- Bright red and pink lipstick will also give the illusion of whiter teeth and will make your smile more alluring.

- Hydrate your lips. Dry, cracked lips look worse with lipstick or gloss. It tends to magnify that they are dry. When you smile, you want your lips to be soft and hydrated for the prettiest smile. See the sidebar on how to get soft, sexy lips.

- Smile with your eyes and mouth. When you smile with your eyes, you appear warm and approachable.

Get Soft, Kissable Lips

Exfoliating and caring for your lips can take you from a Yuck Mouth to a Yes Mouth! Here are four easy steps you can do to get you pucker perfect. Muah!

1. **APPLY LIP BALM BEFORE YOU GO TO SLEEP AT NIGHT.** It will soften the dead skin so it lifts easier. Try Bite Beauty Agave Lip Mask (EWG score: 2) made with only four ingredients.

2. **MIX BROWN SUGAR AND COCONUT OIL INTO A PASTY CONSIS-TENCY.** Then gently rub the mixture in small circular motions to exfoliate the skin. Rinse with warm water. If you don't want to make your own scrub, try Tarte Maracuja Lip Exfoliant (EWG score: 1*), which will do the trick too, and since it's USDA Organic, you don't have to worry if you get a little in your mouth.

3. **SMEAR ON ECO LIPS SOFTENING LIP BALM RELIEVE, COCOA VANILLA** (EWG score: 0*) to moisturize and protect against damaging free radicals. Apply liberally, as there are no harsh chemicals.

GREEN BEAUTY SECRET NO. 10: HAVE CONFIDENCE

Above all, do this! Have confidence. This is your biggest secret weapon, even before concealer. The way you feel directly impacts the way you look. Having confidence will help you look and feel gorgeous. You can pull off just about any look you want if you are feeling it. The confidence you have will carry the look. I have seen beauty looks that make a Picasso painting look like realism, and still I have found them shockingly beautiful because they were worn with so much confidence; they owned it.

Vivian Diller, a psychologist and the author of *Face It*, interviewed hundreds of women and found that the most frequent comment she heard from them was that beauty is about confidence. She said she learned this early on from Wilhelmina Cooper, founder of Wilhelmina Models, where she modeled in the 1970s. Cooper said, "The chances of booking work for us rises the minute you take on an air of confidence, no matter what you look like."[13] She goes on to say that holding your head up high with poise and confidence is probably the number one quality that women say leads to feeling and looking beautiful at any age. Amen!

So what if you don't have confidence? Cultivate it! Confidence doesn't necessarily happen overnight. It's a process that you will need to practice. We all have self-doubt sometimes, but with confidence, you can overcome it. Here are some simple tools you can use to help build self-confidence.

1. **MIND YOUR MANNERS.** Confidence shows in many ways: your posture, your behavior, the way you speak, and the things you say. Stand up tall, pull your shoulders back, hold your head up

high, smile, and make eye contact. Act confident, even if you don't feel confident.

2. **LOOK THE PART.** Dress for confidence and focus on your good qualities. Do you have legs that would make Naomi Campbell jealous? Play them up. Wear a short skirt or long slit that lets your leg peek through à la Angelina Jolie on the red carpet. If you have a long, graceful neck, show it. Pull your hair back and wear fabulous earrings to showcase it and draw attention. Being well groomed and looking good will boost self-confidence. Spend some time on yourself and pay attention to personal hygiene.

3. **THINK ABOUT YOUR STRENGTHS AND TALENTS.** Recognize your good qualities and what you have already achieved. You will feel good knowing you have strong character, can do something well, or can master something that you've put your mind to. Having a sense of self-efficiency will boost your self-esteem, a quality that is high in confident people.

4. **THINK POSITIVE.** Positive people tend to feel better about themselves and others. Try not to dwell on the problems in your life; instead focus on solutions and making positive changes. Stop negative thoughts as they pop into your head and replace them with positive ones. Mantras are great. Repeat positive messages to yourself. It works.

Chapter Nine

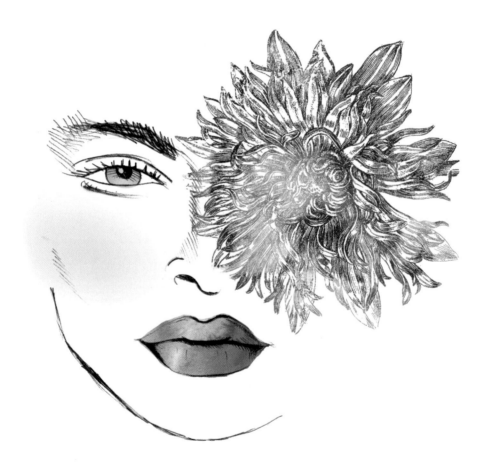

Green Beauty
Looks

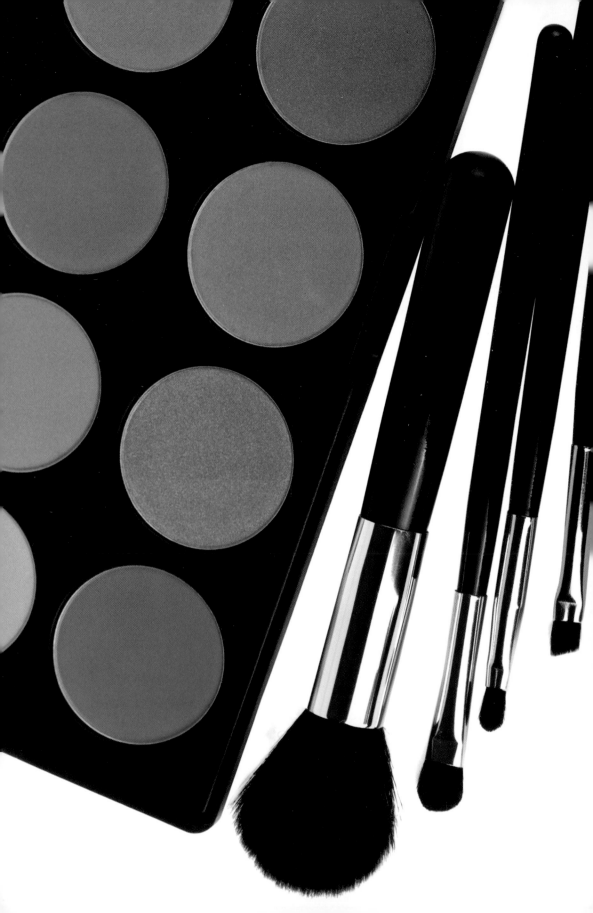

Creating beautiful, wearable looks with chemically safe makeup is no different from creating them with traditional, premium, or designer brand cosmetics. It's all about technique and knowing how to work with the textures. I created these wearable beauty looks from natural to bold using chemically safe and natural brands. The looks are easy to recreate at home and hopefully will inspire you to be a little daring and experiment with different looks. Go ahead, be fabulous!

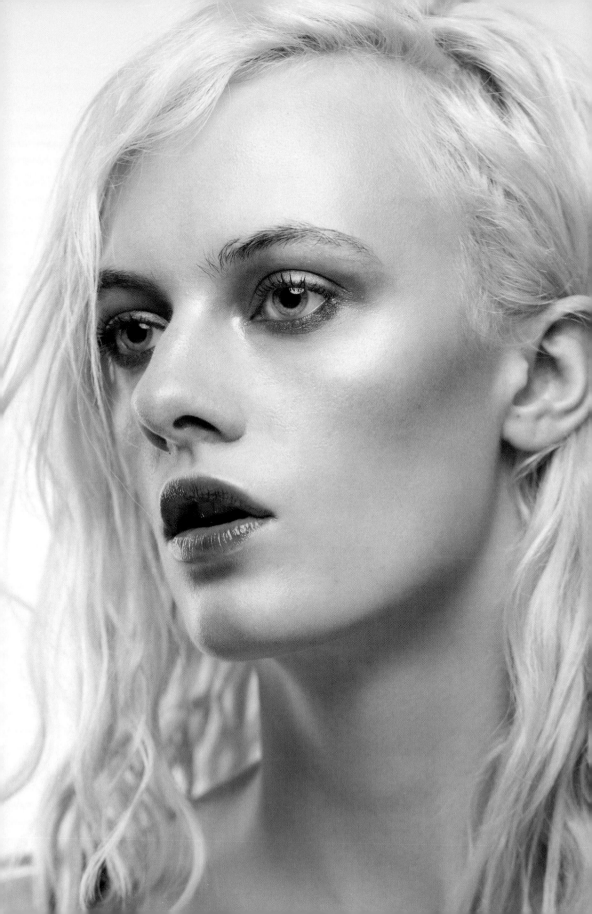

BRONZED

Green Beauty Products Used	EWG Ranking
W3ll People Narcissist Foundation + Concealer No 2	2*
Antonym Baked Blush Copper	2*
Antonym Quattro Croisette Eyeshadow Bark	2*
DeVita Absolute Minerals Softlines Eyeliner Pencil Earth	2*
Mineral Fusion Sheer Moisture Lip Tints Smolder	2*
RMS Beauty Living Luminizer	1
Antonym Certified Natural Lola Lash Mascara Black	2*
W3ll People Realist Invisible Setting Powder	1*
Beautycounter Color Define Brow Pencil Light	0

Asterisks indicate products not found in EWG's database; scored using Build Your Own Report tool.

Step-by-Step Guide: *Bronzed*

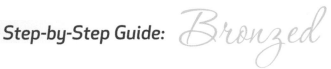

1. **FOUNDATION /CONCEALER:** Using a concealer brush, I spot touched concealer/foundation on the face where needed covering any redness or dark spots.

   ✦ **Pro Tip:** *To get the shiny gritty look I wanted, I left her skin very sheer and well hydrated. A flawless matte finish would take away from that.*

2. **BLUSH:** Using an angled blush brush, I applied the blush just along the cheek bone with a heavy hand. I wanted a bronzed look that's heated looking and fiery. Not a tan look but more of a summer beauty look.

3. **EYEBROWS:** I lightly defined the brows with a blonde pencil for more shape.

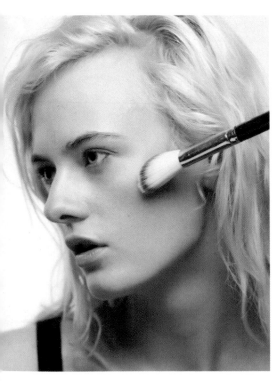
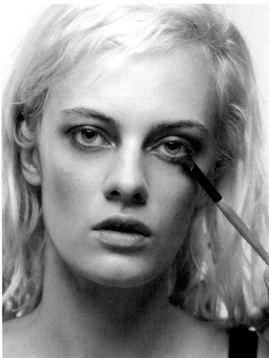

4. EYE SHADOW: Using a medium fluffy eye shadow brush, I applied the shadow to the eyelids and under the eye using a small, round eye shadow brush.

5. EYELINER: I lined the waterline with a soft brown eyeliner on the bottom only.

6. LASHES: I curled Erika's lashes and applied one coat of mascara.

7. LIPSTICK: I drew on a sheer candy apple lip tint.

8. POWDER: Using a powder brush, I lightly dusted powder around her nose and lip area.

9. HIGHLIGHTER: I applied an illuminator down the bridge of the nose and on top of the cheek bones to give the look extra shine and hot spots.

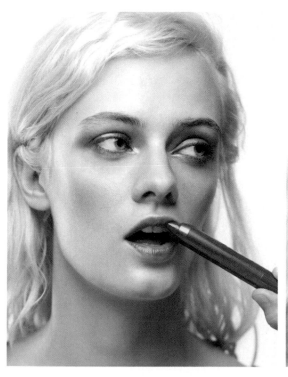
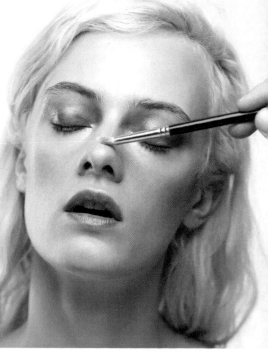

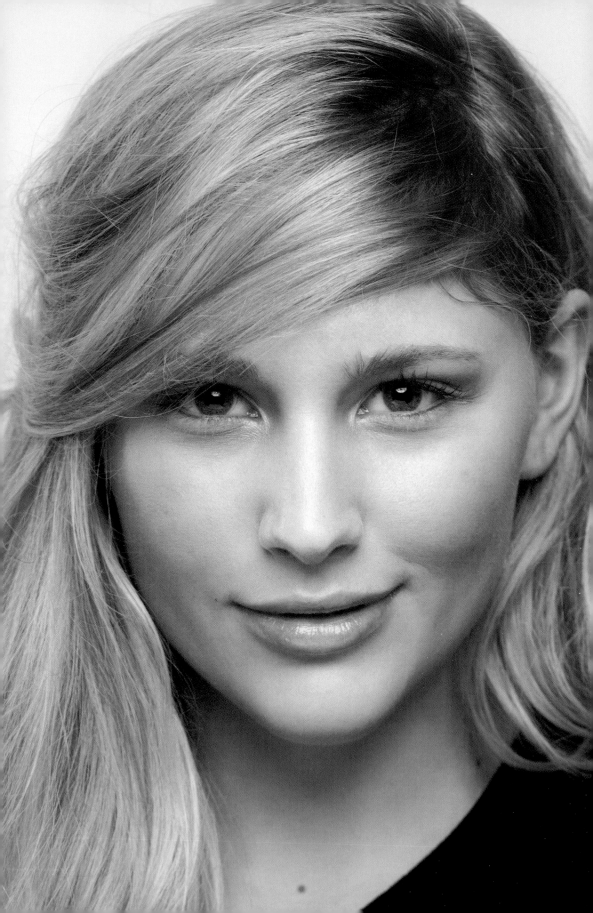

NATURAL

Green Beauty Products Used	EWG Ranking
RMS Beauty "Un" Cover-Up, Shade 11	1
W3ll People Realist Invisible Setting Powder	1*
Beautycounter Color Shade Eye Duo, Shell/Malt	1
Beautycounter Color Lip, Sheer Nude	1
Inika Certified Organic Eyeliner, Coco	2
Beautycounter Color Sweep Blush Duo, Tawny/Whisper	1
Gabriel Cosmetics Mascara, Black	2

Asterisks indicate products not found in EWG's database; scored using Build Your Own Report tool.

Step-by-Step Guide: *Natural*

1. **CONCEALER:** I applied concealer under Liberty's eyes and around her nose and spot treated any areas that needed it. This is not a polished look but rather relaxed and no fuss, so there is no need to apply foundation to the entire face.

   ✦ **Pro Tip:** *Use your concealer brush to swipe over the eyelids to give extra brightening.*

2. **POWDER:** I dusted her entire face with a light coat of setting powder, concentrating on the areas where I used concealer.

   ✦ **Pro Tip:** *Use powder only in the T-zone area if you prefer a more dewy finish.*

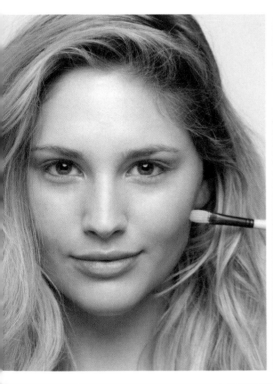
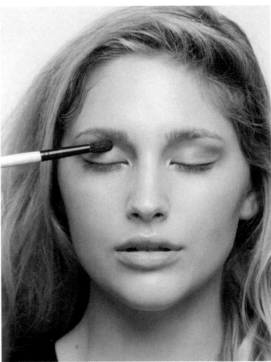

3. **EYE SHADOW:** I swept pale pink color over the entire eyelid, wrapping it around to the bottom lash line. Next, I swiped the warm brown in the crease using both colors in the duo.

4. **EYELINER:** I drew a thin brown line on the bottom lash line just halfway, stopping in the middle.

5. **BLUSH:** I swirled the orange-brown blush on the apples of her cheeks, sweeping back toward the hairline.

6. **LIPSTICK:** I painted her lips with the sheer nude color using a lip brush.

7. **LASHES:** Last, I applied one coat of black mascara.

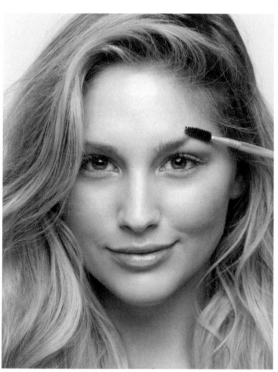
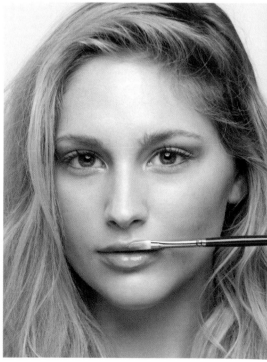

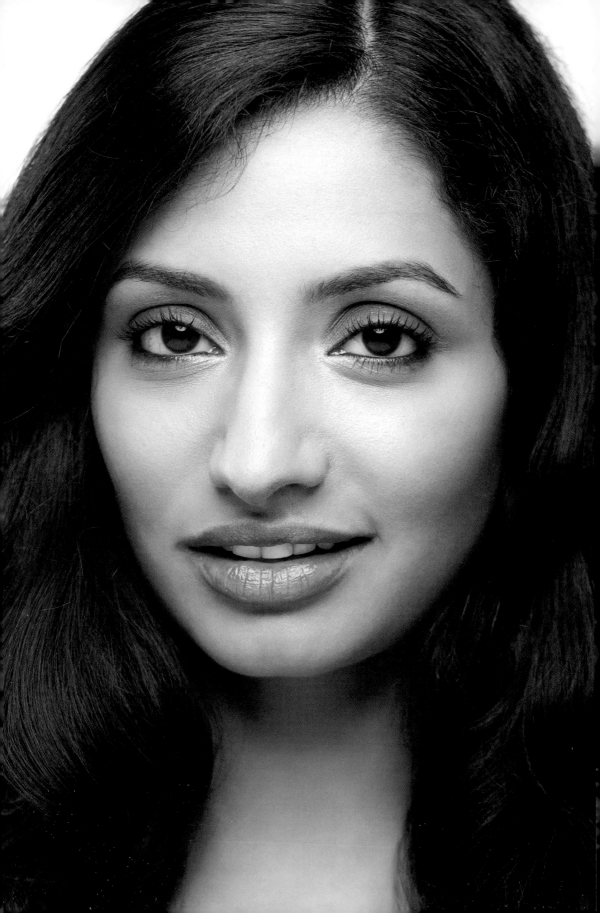

GLAMOROUS

Green Beauty Products Used	EWG Ranking
Vapour Organic Beauty Atmosphere Luminous Foundation 140	2*
RMS Beauty "Un" Cover-Up 33	1*
Beautycounter Color Define Brow Pencil Medium	0
W3ll People Bio Bronzer Natural Tan	1*
Inika Mineral Blush Peachy Keen	1*
Kjaer Weis Eyeshadow Green Depth	2*
Jane Iredale 24-Karat Gold Dust	2*
GlamNatural Eye Pencil Black Opal	1* (one unknown ingredient)
Kjaer Weis Lip Tint Sweetness	3*
W3ll People Bio Brightener Invisible Powder	3*
W3ll People Expressionist Bio Extreme Mascara in Black	3

Asterisks indicate products not found in EWG's database; scored using Build Your Own Report tool.

Step-by-Step Guide: *Glamorous*

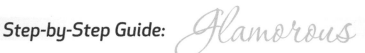

1. **FOUNDATION:** I smoothed on foundation starting in the T-zone, working my way down the neck and chest to match the face.

2. **CONCEALER:** I dabbed on concealer from the inner corner to the outer corner, blending with a clean, soft eye shadow brush.

3. **EYESHADOW:** I layered the green shadow over the eyelid from the lash line to the crease with a large eye shadow brush. Then I popped the inner corners with the gold dust, using a small, round eye shadow brush.

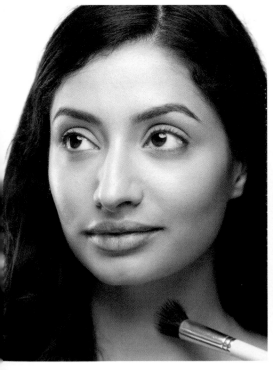
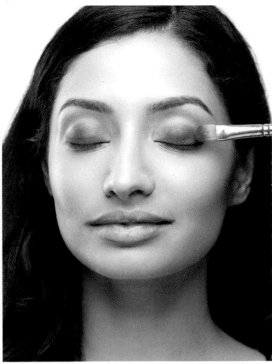

4. **EYELINER:** Using a black pencil, I lined the upper lash line and waterline on the top and bottom.

   ✦ **Pro Tip:** *Warm up a freshly sharpened pencil on the back of your hand by drawing a few lines before using. It will go on easier.*

5. **EYE BROWS:** I defined the entire brow with a medium brown brow pencil.

6. **BLUSH:** Starting on the apples of the cheek, I swept on the peach blush.

7. **LIP TINT:** Using a lip brush, I patted on a tangerine lip tint.

8. **LASHES:** After curling the lashes, I coated them twice with mascara.

9. **POWDER:** I finished the look with a brightening powder under the eyes and around the nose and mouth.

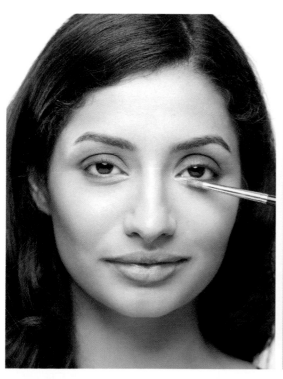
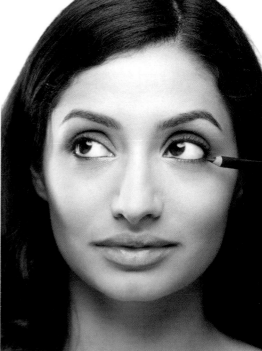

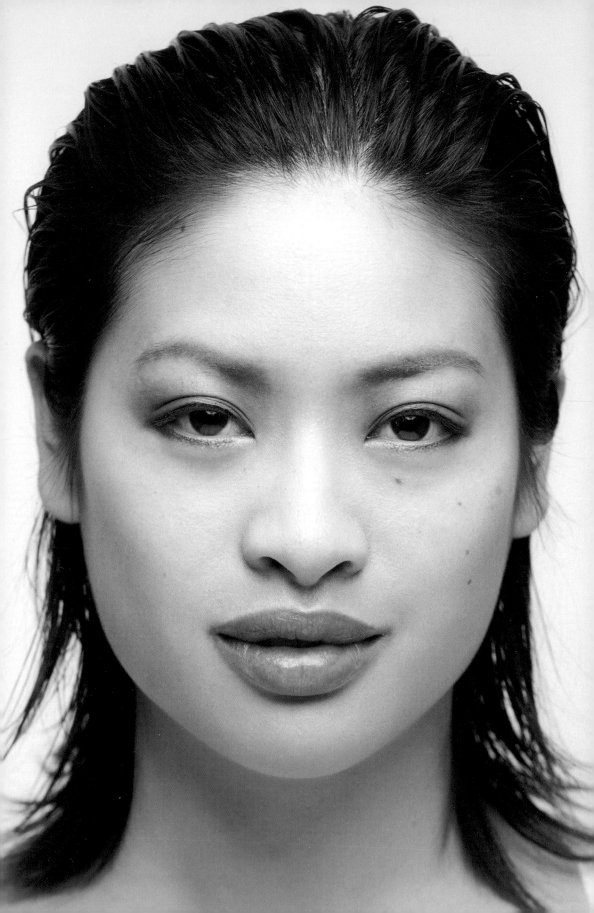

BOLD

Green Beauty Products Used	EWG Ranking
W3ll People Narcissist Foundation Stick, No. 3	2
Zuii Organic Flora Powder Foundation, Ivory	1*
W3ll People Universalist Multi-use Color Stick, No. 8	2*
Kjaer Weis Eye Shadow, Blue Wonder	1*
GlamNatural Eye Shadow, Cocoa Mauve	2*
Mineral Fusion Sheer Moisture Lip Tint, Glisten	2*
ZuZu Luxe Brow Pencil, Russet	2*
Ilia Complete Mascara, Macao	1*
Jane Iredale Liquid Eyeliner, Black	1
W3ll People Expressionist Bio Extreme Mascara, Black	3

Asterisks indicate products not found in EWG's database; scored using Build Your Own Report tool.

Step-by-Step Guide 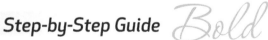 *Bold*

1. **FOUNDATION/CONCEALER:** Using a concealer brush, I applied concealer/foundation to the center of the face around the nose and chin, blending outward to the hairline. I did not cover the entire face as Jennifer has great skin and it wasn't needed. I spot treated the face where needed by covering any redness or dark spots.

2. **BLUSH:** Using a synthetic foundation brush, I applied the cream blush in the way I would a contour. I wanted the focus to be on the eyes instead of competing with the blush. I chose a peachy color and blended with my fingertips.

✦ **Pro Tip:** *Synthetic brushes work well for cream products as they do not absorb the product the way a natural bristle brush does.*

3. POWDER: Using a powder brush, I lightly dusted powder only over the areas where I used concealer/foundation to take down any shine, concentrating on the T-zone.

4. EYEBROWS: I filled in the brows with a pencil a couple of shades lighter than Jennifer's natural brows but only where they were sparse. I then brushed through a bronze-colored mascara to tone them down. I wanted a softer eyebrow so the color really popped. I wanted them to be groomed and polished but, again, not the focal point.

5. EYELINER: I lined the upper lid with a black liquid liner, keeping it extremely close to the lash line to create some definition, but I didn't want to see it; I only wanted to see the color. For the lower lashes, I used a chocolate brown shadow to create a clean

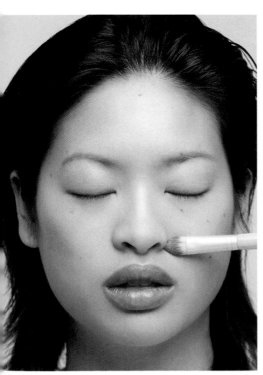
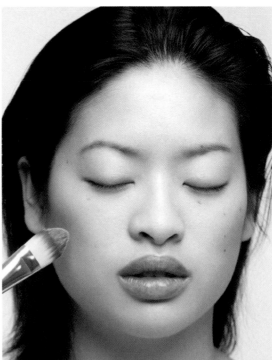

line on the lower lashes. I drew from the outer corner inward, not quite connecting the line to the inner corner.

6. EYE SHADOW: I used a medium fluffy shadow brush to apply the blue eye shadow to the eyelid, blending beyond the crease and into the lash line. I softened any hard edges using my fingertip.

  ✦ **Pro Tip:** *It doesn't need to be precise—I prefer a more organic eye. The result is pretty but not too "done" looking.*

7. MASCARA: I skipped the curler for the model's lashes, opting for straighter lashes, and applied one coat of black mascara.

8. LIPSTICK: Last, I drew on a salmon-hued lipstick. It's a sheer and shiny lipstick that can't go wrong. I preferred the sheer texture with all the color on the eyes.

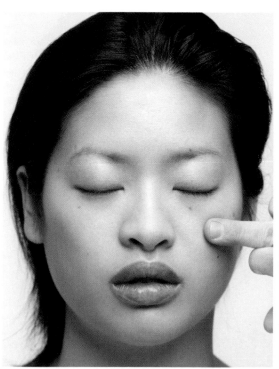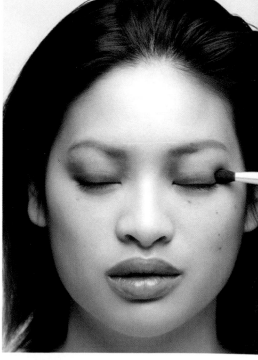

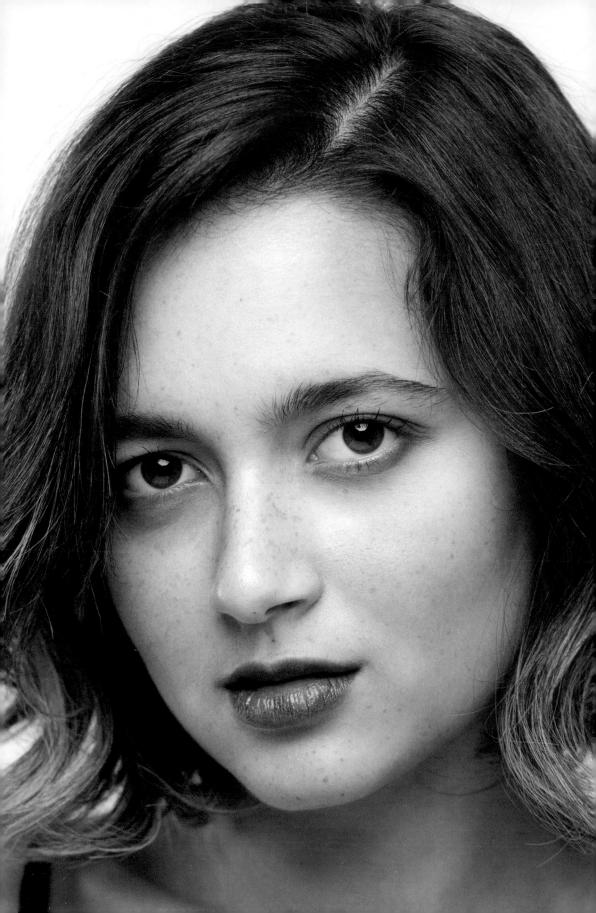

FLUSHED

Green Beauty Products Used	EWG Ranking
Tarte Maracuja Creasless Concealer Tan	2
W3ll People Realist Invisible Setting Powder	1*
Tarte Amazonian Clay 12 Hour Blush Frisky	3
Tarte Eye Shadow Dreamer	2
Kjaer Weis Lip Tint Goddess	3*
W3ll People Expressionist Bio Extreme Mascara Black	3

Asterisks indicate products not found in EWG's database; scored using Build Your Own Report tool.

Step-by-Step Guide: 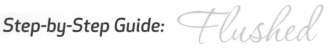 *Flushed*

1. **CONCEALER:** I spot treated the areas of the face that needed coverage and concealed under the eyes.

2. **EYESHADOW:** I washed shadow over her lids to the crease to enhance her skin's natural color with a fluffy round blender brush.

3. **BLUSH:** I flushed Camille's cheeks by using a stipple blush brush starting on the apples of the cheek and sweeping slightly down and toward the hairline to mimic a natural flush.

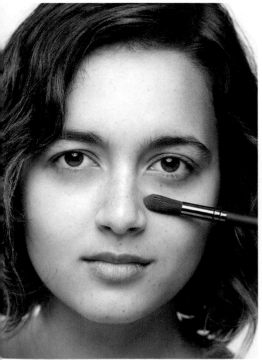 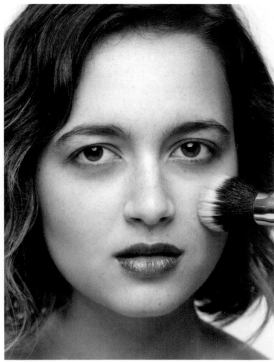

4. **LIPSTICK:** Next I generously painted her lips with burgundy colored lip tint with a lip brush and then had her blot on a tissue to leave a stain.

5. **LASHES:** I applied one coat of black mascara to keep the eyes subdued.

6. **POWDER:** I dusted the T-zone area to take down any shine.

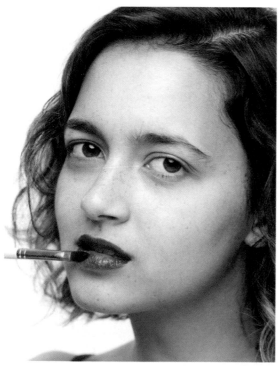
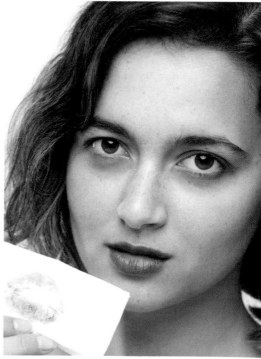

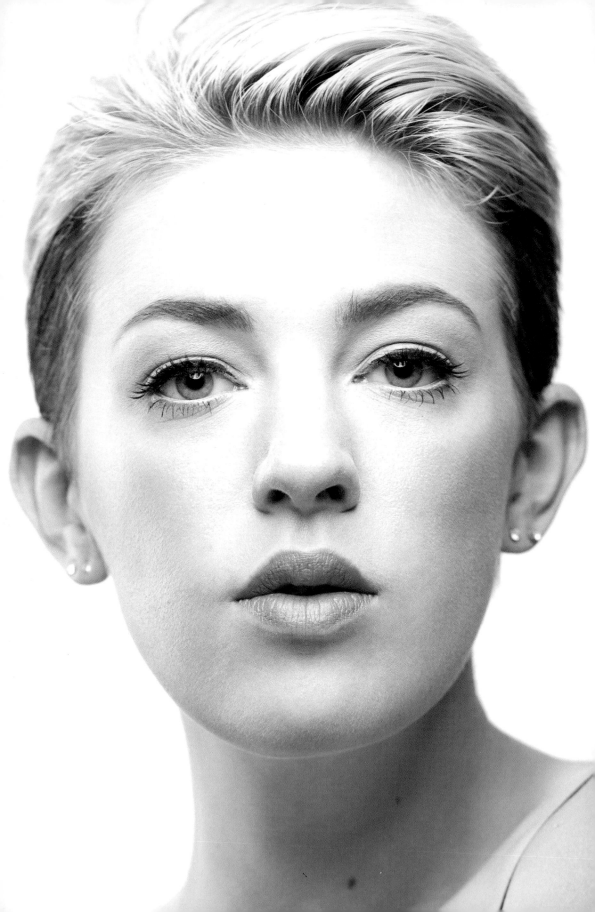

GAMINE

Green Beauty Products Used	EWG Ranking
Zuii Organic Certified Organic Foundation Primer	1*
Kjaer Weis Foundation Paper Thin	1*
Zuii Organic Certified Organic Eye Shadow Chestnut	1*
Zuzu Luxe Brow Pencil Blonde	2*
Dr. Hauschka Eyeliner Duo Gray/White	3
Jane Iredale Liquid Eyeliner Black	1
Tata Harper Volumizing Lip and Cheek Tint Very Popular	3
Antonym Certified Natural Lola Lash Mascara Black	2*
W3ll People Realist Invisible Setting Powder	1*
Georgie Clear Faux Lash Adhesive	3*

Asterisks indicate products not found in EWG's database; scored using Build Your Own Report tool.

Step-by-Step Guide: *Jamine*

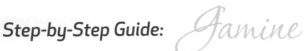

1. **PREP:** To create a smooth matte finish I applied primer to Raye's face.

2. **FOUNDATION:** Using a synthetic rounded, flat foundation brush, I applied the foundation to her entire face, blending into the ears and hairline.

3. **BLUSH:** Using my fingers, I pressed cream lip and cheek tint on the apples of the cheek and then blended with a stippled blush brush to give a seamless pop of color.

4. **EYE SHADOW:** I washed the eye shadow across the crease with a large fluffy blender brush.

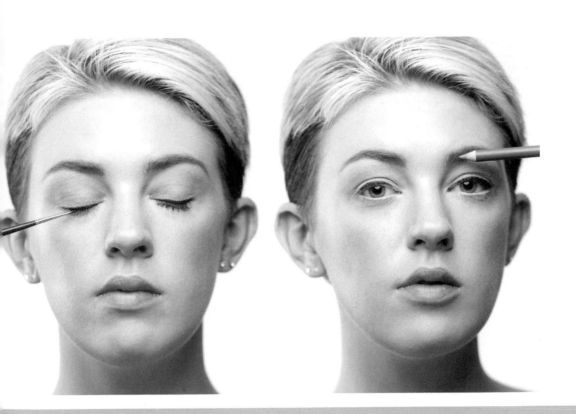

5. **EYELINER:** With black liquid liner, I drew a thin line on the top lash line. I lined the waterline with white pencil.

6. **EYEBROWS:** I created definition and fuller brows using a blonde pencil.

7. **LIPSTICK:** To create pouty lips, I patted the lip and cheek tint onto the center of the lips, blending to the edges.

9. **LASHES:** After curling her lashes, I topped them with two coats of black mascara and spikey strip lashes.

✦ **Pro Tip:** *Using an eyeliner brush, line the lash line with eyelash glue and then press on the lashes.*

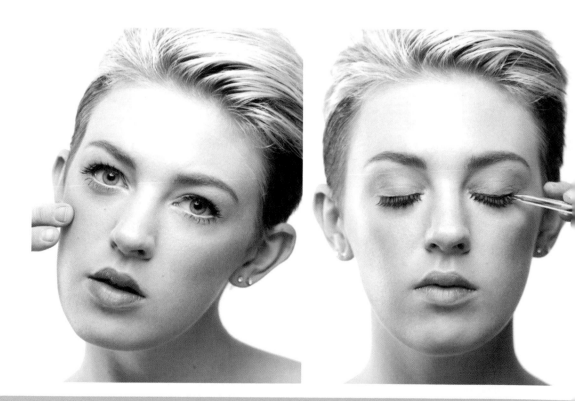

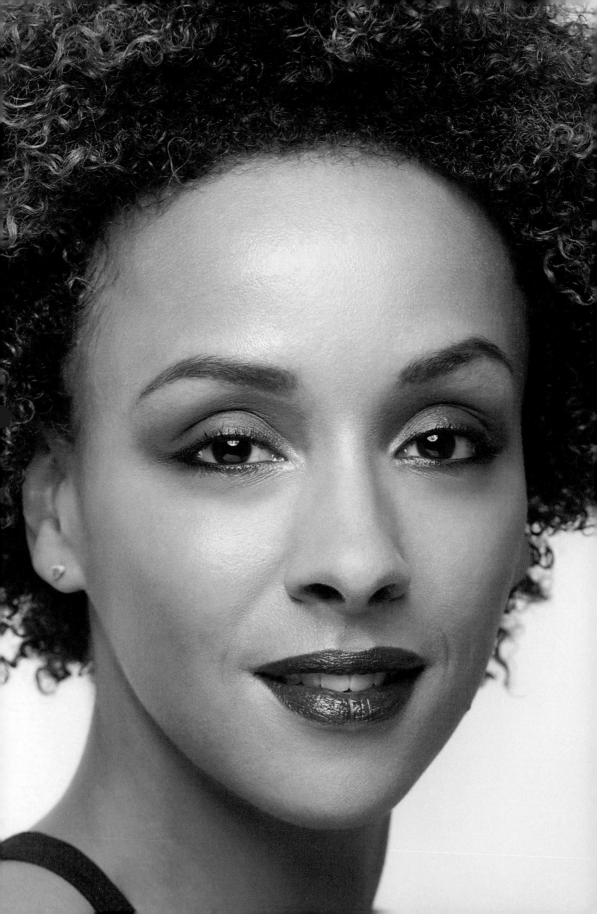

CHIC

Green Beauty Products Used	EWG Ranking
Zuii Organic Certified Organic Foundation Primer	1*
Kjaer Weis Cream Foundation, Velvety	1*
GlamNatural Mineral Eye Shadow, Fresh Berries	2*
Jane Iredale Eyeliner Pencil, Basic Black	1
GlamNatural Mineral Brow Pencil, Medium Brown	1
Gabriel Cosmetics Multi Pot, Florentina	0*
Primitive Natural Lip Pencil, Martinique	1
Ilia Lipstick, Ink Pot	2
W3ll People, Expressionist Bio Extreme Mascara	3

*Asterisks indicate products not found in EWG's database; scored using Build Your Own Report tool.

Step-by-Step Guide *Chic*

1. **PREP:** I prepped Michelle's skin with a primer to control oil, applying it over the entire face.

2. **FOUNDATION:** I applied the cream foundation to her entire face starting at the center and moving outward, blending into the hairline and ears and down the neck.

3. **BLUSH:** Using my fingers, I lightly patted the cream blush on the apples of her cheeks and blended well. I wanted this look to be sophisticated, so I kept everything in the same tones—plums and berries.

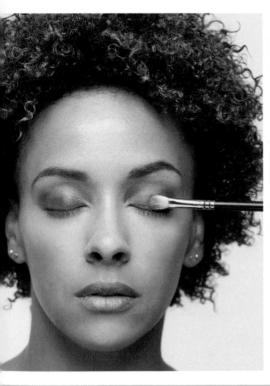
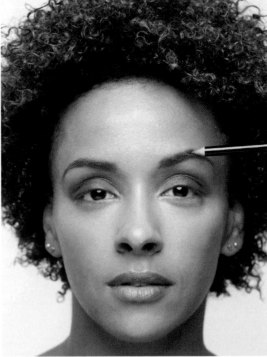

4. **EYE SHADOW:** Next, I washed a berry shadow across the eyelid with a medium shadow brush, elongating the outer corner a bit. I kept the edges soft and sheer.

5. **EYELINER:** With black liner, I lined the top and bottom lids close to the lash line and then blended it with a smudge brush.

6. **EYEBROWS:** I groomed the brows with a medium brown pencil only where needed.

7. **LIPSTICK:** To define the lips, I first lined them with a violet brown liner, leaving the center of the bottom lip clean to create a highlight, then topped it with a violet lipstick.

✦ **Pro Tip:** *For staying power, fill in the entire lip with a matching pencil and then apply the lipstick.*

8. **LASHES:** After curling her lashes, I topped them with two coats of mascara.

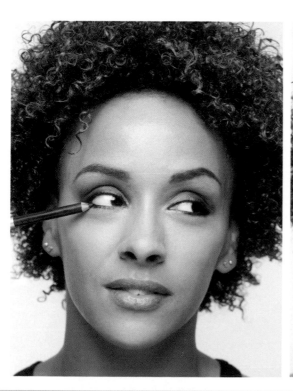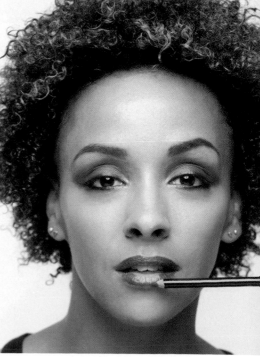

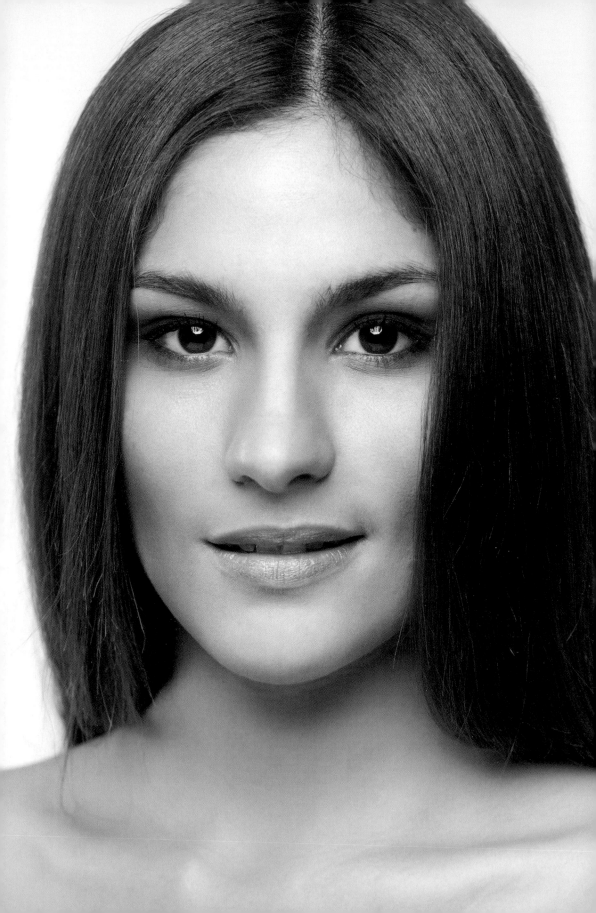

SULTRY

Green Beauty Products Used	EWG Ranking
Jane Iredale Smooth Affair Facial Primer & Brightener	2
Jane Iredale Liquid Minerals Foundation, Latte	2
Ecco Bella FlowerColor Cover Up	3
Ecco Bella FlowerColor Face Powder, Medium	2
Jane Iredale Jelly Jar, Black	1*
Gabriel Eye Shadow Trio, Smokey & Classic	2*
Ecco Bella FlowerColor Bronzing Powder	2
Beautycounter Lip Sheer, Twig	1

*Asterisks indicate products not found in EWG's database; scored using Build Your Own Report tool.

Step-by-Step Guide: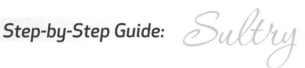

1. **PREP:** I prepped the skin with a primer to create a smooth canvas.

2. **CONCEALER:** Next, I applied concealer underneath the eyes at the inner corners and spot treated the face.

3. **FOUNDATION:** I swirled on foundation to the entire face, keeping it very sheer and natural looking.

   ✦ **Pro Tip:** *Use a round, soft foundation brush or a stipple brush to break up the minerals for a seamless application.*

4. **EYELINER:** Using a smudger brush, I smudged in gel eyeliner at the base of her top lashes and blended it into the lid.

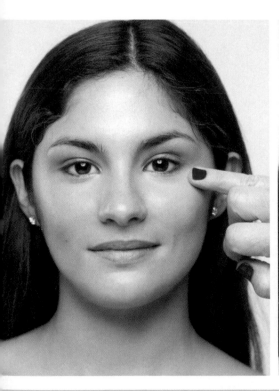
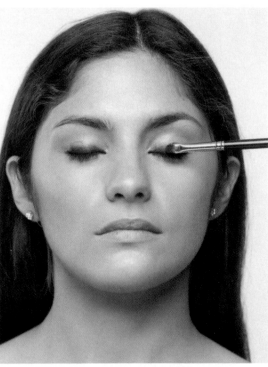

5. **EYE SHADOW:** I layered the charcoal gray color over the liner up to the crease and onto the bottom lash line. In the crease, I used a warm brown for contour and blended it all together with a blending brush. Last, I dusted the cream color under the eyebrows to highlight her brow bone. I prefer a lighter version of the smoky eye, so I kept everything soft and sheer.

6. **BRONZER/CONTOUR:** I warmed up her face with bronzer, using it as a contour around the edges of her temple, jawline, and under her cheekbones.

7. **POWDER:** I finished her face with a light dusting of powder to create an airbrushed look.

8. **LIPSTICK:** I completed her look with a coat of lipstick for a nude, sheer lip.

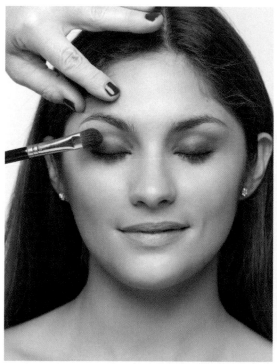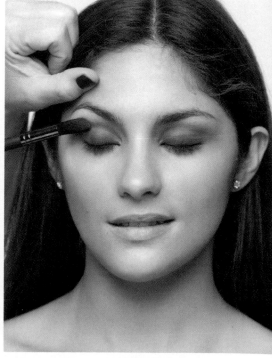

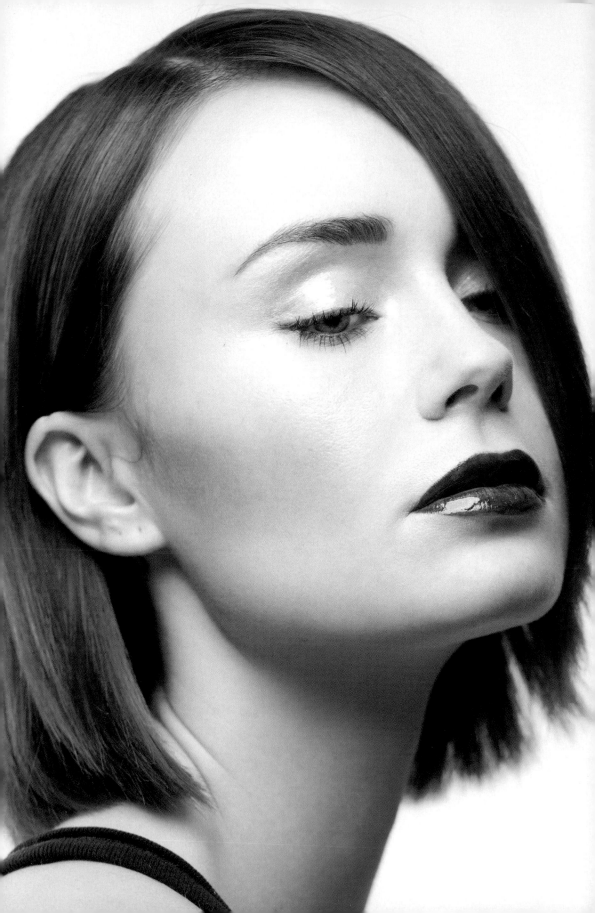

CLASSIC

Green Beauty Products Used	EWG Ranking
Zuzu Luxe Oil Free Liquid Foundations L-6	3
Tarte Maracuja Creasless Concealer Fair	2
W3ll People Realist Invisible Setting Powder	1*
Jane Iredale Eye Gloss Liquid Eye Shadow Champagne	1
Jane Iredale PurePressed Eye Shadow Taupe	1
Jane Iredale Lip Definer Berry	1
Jane Iredale PureMoist Lipstick Annette	1*
Jane Iredale Lip Fixation Cherish (gloss only)	1*
Antonym Certified Natural Lola Lash Mascara Black	2*
Ecco Bella FlowerColor Blush Nutmeg	3

Asterisks indicate products not found in EWG's database; scored using Build Your Own Report tool.

Step-by-Step Guide: 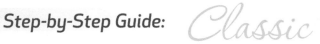 *Classic*

1. **FOUNDATION:** I brushed on foundation over the entire face, blending it with a clean, fluffy kabuki brush for a flawless finish.

2. **CONCEALER:** I concealed under the eyes and around the nose.

3. **POWDER:** I set her foundation by lightly dusting her face with a coat of finishing powder.

4. **EYE SHADOW:** I swiped on a thin layer of liquid eye shadow using a medium eye shadow brush to the eyelid. On the bottom lash line, I applied the taupe shadow with a small round eye-shadow brush.

   ✦ **Pro Tip:** *Fingers work just as well for liquid eye shadow.*

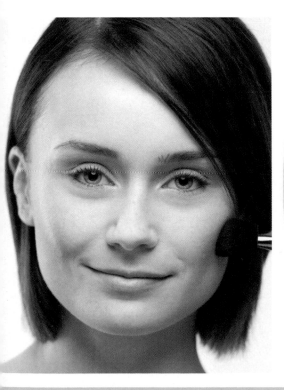
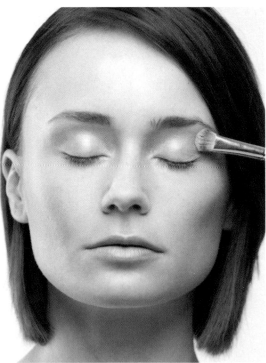

5. **BLUSH:** I used the blush as a contour. Using a flat contour brush, I concentrated the color just under her cheekbone.

6. **LIPSTICK:** Using a lip brush, I painted her lips with the lipstick.

7. **LIP LINER:** Next, I lined her lips with the lip pencil.

8. **LIP GLOSS:** I topped her lips with a clear gloss.

9. **LASHES:** Finally, I applied one coat of black mascara.

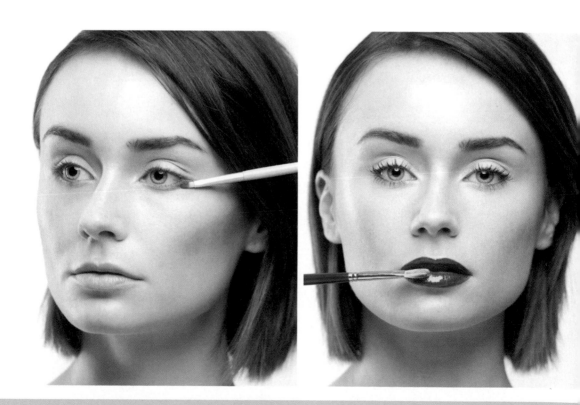

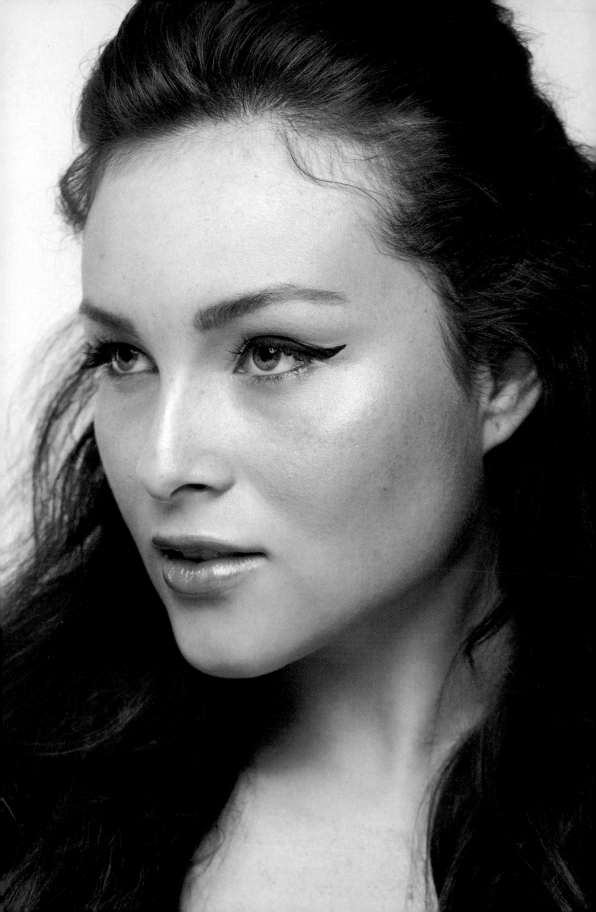

FLIRTY

Green Beauty Products Used	EWG Ranking
Beautycounter Tint Skin Foundation, Linen	2*
ZuZu Luxe Liquid Eyeliner, Raven	3
Beautycounter Touchup Skin Concealer Pen	1
ZuZu Luxe Eye Shadow, Chameleon	2
Inika Certified Organic Brow Pencil, Brunette Beauty	1
Zuii Organic Certified Organic Flora Blush, Melon	2*
RMS Beauty Living Luminizer	1
Jane Iredale PureGloss Lip Gloss, Nectar	1
Gabriel Cosmetics Mascara, Black	2

Asterisks indicate products not found in EWG's database; scored using Build Your Own Report tool.

Step-by-Step Guide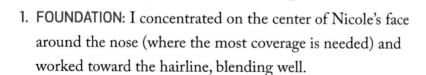

1. **FOUNDATION:** I concentrated on the center of Nicole's face around the nose (where the most coverage is needed) and worked toward the hairline, blending well.

2. **EYEBROWS:** I used a brow pencil in a brunette shade that closely matched the natural brow color. I brushed them up using a spoolie brush and then swept them across to lie naturally.

3. **EYELINER:** This look is all about the eyeliner. Using a thin liner brush and liquid liner, I drew a thick, elongated line from the outer corner to the middle of the lash line, and then started at the inner corner and drew a line to the middle of the lash line to connect the two lines. I went over it a few times until the line

was the thickness and angle I wanted. You don't have to be as dramatic with the line. A little flick on the outer corners may be all you need. I like to use my own brush, so I place the product on the back of my hand and use it as my palette. It keeps my hands free to work and the liner close by.

✦ **Pro Tip:** *If you need to clean up the line, use a little oil or moisturizer on a cosmetic remover swab or smudger brush to remove mistakes. Then follow up with concealer.*

4. **EYE SHADOW:** Using a large, fluffy blender brush, I swept the bronze brown eye shadow over the crease of the eye to create depth. The crease is diffused. It's not a dark, defined line.

5. **CONCEALER:** I used a concealer pen to touch up the inner corners of the eye and underneath, covering any blue, red, or purple tones.

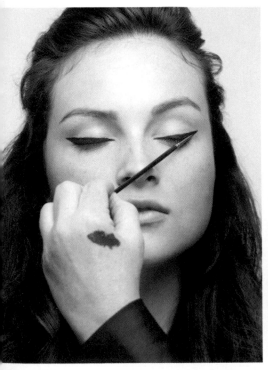
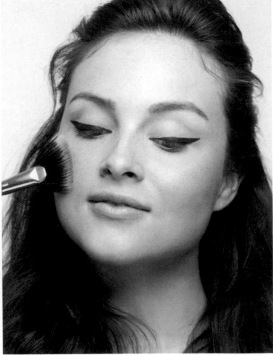

6. **HIGHLIGHTER:** Next, I lightly tapped on a cream illuminizer on the top of the cheekbone using a concealer brush.

7. **BLUSH:** Using a fan brush, I swept a hint of the peachy pink color on the apples of the cheeks. This is not a blushing look; I just added a whisper of color for radiance.

8. **LASHES:** I curled her lashes and then applied three coats of black mascara.

9. **LIP GLOSS:** Finally, I brushed on apricot-colored gloss with a lip brush for an über feminine look that's not tough. This look would work well with a matte lipstick too.

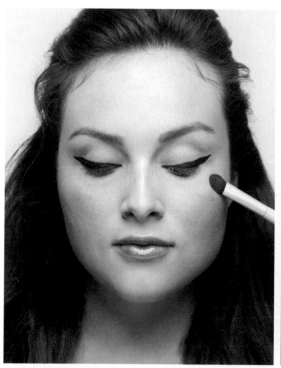
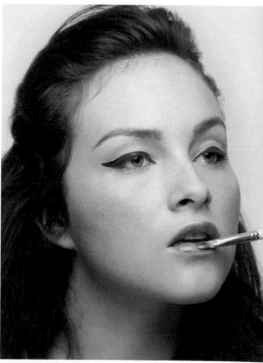

How to Take the Best Selfies Ever

We are a culture obsessed with selfies. They may seem a bit cheesy, but we are all guilty of taking them, so why not own it? Stars aren't the only ones who can look amazing in selfies. Here's how you can look your personal best.

Makeup check. Add some definition to your face. Apply color to your lips and cheeks and line your eyes. A camera flash can wash you out. Take down any shine with blot papers or pressed powder.

Face the light. Never have the light source behind you or overhead, which will create shadows under your eyes.

Angle your body slightly away from the camera; it's more sliming than straight on.

Hold the camera slightly above your head for the most flattering angle.

Hold still, smile, and take a winning picture.

Edit the image. Use an app with fun filters or one that can remove a blemish to create the perfect selfie.

Red Carpet Rules

Snap a picture of yourself using a flash.

Before you leave the house, check for "raccoon eyes," peekaboo clothing, and overall look in general.

Hydrate any skin that shows to give it a glow. Use self-tanner or bronzer if you are pasty.

Use bling sparingly and in the right places.

Do a teeth check. Look for lipstick on the teeth as well as bits of nibbles between your teeth.

Carry concealer, powder, and lipstick for touch-ups; lashes and lash glue if you are wearing lashes; tissue; mirrored compact; and mints.

Mineral Makeup Mistakes Women Make and How to Correct Them

MISTAKE NO. 1: **Applying too much powder foundation.** Powder foundations tend to look cakey and dry. They can also add years to your face.

SOLUTION NO. 1: **Apply a liquid or cream foundation first, then apply the powder lightly.** If you prefer a powder foundation, then spot treat the face with concealer first, then use the powder foundation so you don't have to use as much.

MISTAKE NO. 2: **Using products with mica or using too much mica.** This can leave the face too shiny or give it an ashy white sheen, especially in photos.

SOLUTION NO. 2: **Use formulations with mica in eye shadows and blush but not foundations and powders.** Use it deliberately to create a glow in one area but not all over the face.

MISTAKE NO. 3: **Assuming a product has enough SPF.** It doesn't.

SOLUTION NO. 3: **You will get some protection from the titanium dioxide and zinc, but it's not enough.** It's fine if you are going grocery shopping, but if you are spending hours outside, you need to wear a proper sunscreen of at least SPF 30.

Chapter Ten

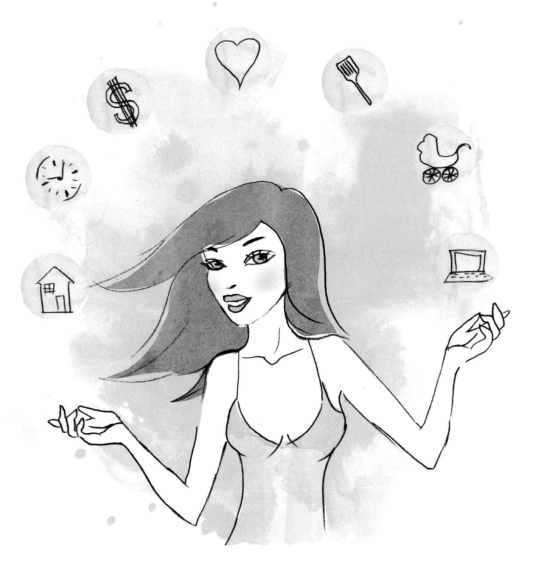

Keeping It
Real

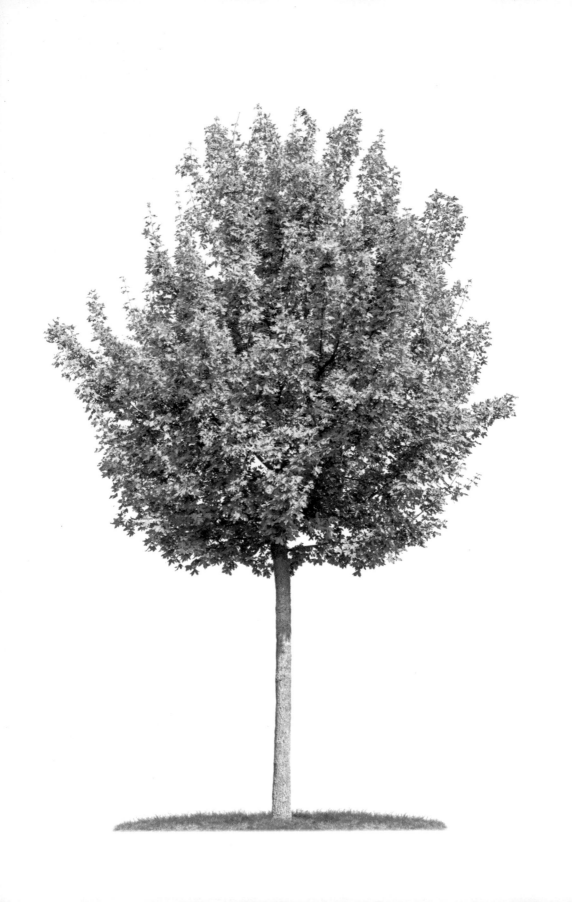

When I heard Ken Cook's talk "Ten Americans" all those years ago, it was a wakeup call. It changed my life. Not only did it change the way I work and the direction of my career, it changed the way I view the world. At the beginning of the book, I mentioned that there is a micro-element and a macro-element approach to toxic cosmetic chemicals. The micro is how it affects you personally. It's about your health. The macro is how it affects the planet and its sustainability. For me, my advocacy started with the macroperspective. I have always had a respect and consciousness for the environment. But Cook's talk opened my eyes to the idea that our earth is a closed circuit. The impact of man-made toxic chemicals on the environment has reached every ecosystem, marine life, tropical region, and the Arctic; they can be found everywhere.[14] Toxic chemicals are endangering our wildlife as well as our own bodies.

For many of you, your journey will start with the microview as you become aware of what these chemicals do to your health. Eventually though, you will see the bigger picture and become concerned with how you and we as a whole are treating our earth. You won't be able to stop it. Once you know the facts, it snowballs. Your awareness becomes keen.

While I was initially concerned with saving the planet, I also wanted to understand how I could step up my eco-efforts in my personal life and career. I realized we need to be equally concerned about our personal health and the health and sustainability of the planet. They are not mutually exclusive. If you harm one, you harm the other. That's when it really clicked for me. We have to be our own advocates. We need to have awareness about what is happening around the world, in our communities, and in our homes.

Now that you have begun the process of greening your beauty routine, I hope you are asking yourself what more you can do. The answer is: a lot! You may not think one person could make a big difference, but you can. Until we don't have to think about it anymore, we have to be our own advocates. One day the cosmetic industry will be regulated. We have a long way to go, but it's starting to slowly happen now. We have yet to pass any federal laws, but it's simply a matter of time before we have a federal policy in place. The pressure is on.

Several states have proposed and adopted cosmetic safety regulations. In 2005, California became the first state in the nation to pass state legislation governing the safety and reporting of cosmetic ingredients. The California Safe Cosmetics Act requires manufacturers to disclose to the state any product ingredient that is on state or federal lists of chemicals that cause cancer or birth defects. In 2008, the state of Washington adopted the Children's Safe Product Act, which requires manufacturers of children's products—including personal care products—sold in Washington to report to the state if their product contains a "Chemical of High Concern to Children."[15] In 2013, Minnesota banned formaldehyde, a cancer-causing chemical, in children's personal care products, such as lotions, shampoos, and bubble baths. The ban against the use of formaldehyde and formaldehyde-releasing preservatives applies to products intended for children under eight.[16]

A CALL TO ACTION

I f you're not already doing so, I urge you help make a change by taking these three simple steps.

1. EMPOWER YOURSELF BY LEARNING AS MUCH AS YOU CAN. Don't stop here. I have merely scratched the surface of the subject. There are so many great books you can read that really dig into the issues concerning toxic chemicals. See the Resources section for some of these.

2. VOTE WITH YOUR DOLLARS. This is the best way to get a company's attention by affecting their bottom line—profits. Buy natural, organic, and chemically safe products, and reject companies that test on animals.

3. GET TO KNOW COSMETIC COMPANIES. Read their mission statements to find out their values. Explore what they stand for and learn about their standards and practices. Get to know what ingredients they use and omit the products that are chemically unsafe. Is the company compassionate to animals and cruelty free? Do they have total transparency? Do they list all their ingredients? You may also want to know if they are on trend and if they come out with new and innovative products. You will soon align with a few of them and be a loyal, lifetime customer.

It's not about being perfect. It's about the process. You are not going to always purchase the healthiest product all the time. You may end up with a product that you love, rather than a product that is healthier for you. No one is going to get it 100 percent right all the time. Nor would I strive to, either. That would be too hard. The green beauty movement has been a slow evolution. We still have to sometimes rely on traditional formulas for certain beauty needs and that's fine, as long as you understand the choices you are making.

Whatever you do, don't feel guilty. You shouldn't feel bad for wanting to feel and look good or wanting luxury and quality goods. I want that, too. It's not about deprivation. No one cares if you purchased your favorite designer fragrance except you—and me. Have I told you how much I love fragrance?

Seriously. I felt guilty for so long and for no good reason. I will tell you a story. Many years ago I had the time to go to green and eco-functions and events. It was a great way to meet like-minded people and get synergy going, not to mention the fact that we had lots of girly fun talking about makeup, skin care, diet, and shoes, of course.

At the time I drove a 2000 Jaguar S-type that I absolutely loved, but I felt incredibly guilty about it. It was a luxury car, after all, and not an eco-friendly one. Before I arrived at the events, I always started to get a bit anxious, wondering if someone would see me pull up in my Jag and would judge me harshly.

It sounds silly now, but it was very real for me at the time. It was so much so that when I arrived at the events, I always parked a couple of blocks away. At the very least, I parked around the block. I didn't want anyone to see me in my Jag. All the other women seemed to drive Priuses. It was so intimidating to drive up to the events and see a sea of Priuses among my big boat especially when there was valet parking. So I stopped doing that early on.

What would happen if they saw me? Would they ban me from the event? Probably not, but I didn't want to find out or hear any judgmental comments. I was in no position to get a new car, even if I wanted to at the time.

One day I outed myself as I so often do. I don't have a lot of secrets. I am pretty much an open book. I was talking to a group of women and someone mentioned something about their SUV, so I called it out. It went something like this. "Phew, I am so glad to hear you drive a Yukon. I drive a Jag, and I was so uncomfortable about it I have been parking blocks away so no one would see me driving it." All the women laughed and said, "No way! We don't care at all; we aren't here to judge you." Then one by one they all started telling on themselves and their not-too-eco-friendly lifestyle choices. One girl even went so far as to make me feel better about driving my Jag. She said it took many more resources to make the Prius than the average car (I'm not sure if that's actually true or not, but I believed it at the time). She praised me for driving a car that was well past five years old and said that that was one of the most environmentally conscious things I could do. It did make me feel better.

I drove my Jag into the ground. After that car, I bought another luxury car—an SUV. I felt good knowing that it was a diesel, so I didn't have any of the guilt I had before. Today I drive a Prius. I love how much money I save on gas and I like the electric element to it. I am a sucker for new technology. Next, I want a Tesla. I can't wait to drive on the superhighway!

I often hear things like, "You would die if you saw what makeup I use," or "Don't judge me," as they smear on a fabulous Chanel lipstick on their lips. I say, "Nah, you should've seen me on Saturday wearing Creed Vetiver fragrance." No judgment here. I get it. I want to look, smell, and feel good too. We are our harshest critics. I beat myself up plenty without having someone else do it. We all want to live healthy, high-quality lives on a thriving, sustainable planet, but that doesn't mean we should be judgmental and critical of others. Want to spread the eco-friendly message with finesse and grace? Here is a little eco-etiquette to help you along the way.

1. LEAD BY EXAMPLE. If you want your family and friends to green their beauty or grooming routine, live a more eco-friendly lifestyle, or be more aware of the chemicals they are coming into contact with in their cosmetics, food, or house-hold products, you must walk the talk. It sends a powerful message to see you making smart purchasing choices or adjustments to your lifestyle.

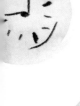

2. DON'T BE JUDGMENTAL. Deliver information in a kind, caring way when there is an opportunity or when you are asked. When you come from a genuine, helpful place, the message is always better received than when it comes from anger or judgment. Don't shove your opinion down someone's throat or take a righteous position. No one likes an overbearing person who is preachy or tries to make you feel stupid. Instead of giving your opinion, share statistical information if the opportunity presents itself. It's hard to negate the World Health Organization.

3. SHARE PRODUCTS AND YOUR TIME. By gifting a product you love to a friend or family member, you may be helping them on their own green beauty journey. It's hard to make the switch when you don't know what you are missing. Offer to shop with them or clean out their products, or teach them how to use a new product. Whether you are sharing a product or your time, your friend or family member will appreciate it.

Finally, I encourage you to strive to live a more sustainable and ultimately healthier lifestyle. Consider your overall chemical exposure. Toxic chemicals are all around us; there is no escaping them, but you can limit your exposure. Try to reduce exposure in all aspects of your life. Eat organic when you can, rid your household cleaning products and detergents of toxic chemicals, clear out toxic household fragrances, such as those found in diffusers, candles, and air fresheners, and buy chemically safe toys and baby gear.

Go deeper with your advocacy. What are you passionate about? Love animals? Volunteer at a shelter. Want your child to have healthier food options at school? Start a petition. Is nature your thing? Help an organization plant trees. Take one small step toward making a change. It doesn't have to be grand or majorly time-consuming. It can be as small as signing a petition or donating money or as big as volunteering your time or starting your own advocacy group. My favorite anthropologist, Jane Goodall, sums it up nicely: "You cannot get through a single day without having an impact on the world around you. What you do makes a difference, and you have to decide what kind of difference you want to make."

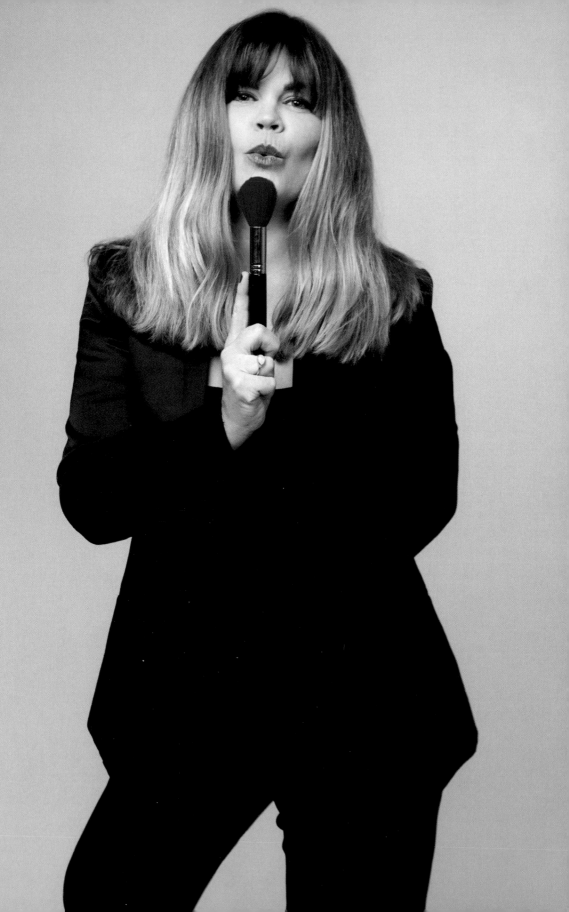

Acknowledgments

Many people were instrumental in the writing of this book. Just as no one really ever raises a child on their own, no author really writes a book on their own. First there are the many people who have talked it out, read over, proofread, written, edited, and designed. Then there are the supporting and encouraging people around you that make the process a bit more manageable. It's a team effort and I am deeply grateful for each and every one of you.

To my daughter, Marianna, you are my inspiration for all I do—you are everything. Thank you for choosing me to be your mommy. I love you endlessly. Thank you to my mom, Diane, and dad, Jim, for making me who I am and always encouraging me to follow my heart—the child with the big dreams. Thank you so much understanding that I needed to see the world. Leaving home wasn't leaving you.

To my stellar literary agent, Steve Harris, thank you for believing in the book from the start. Your humor and clever guidance made this book possible. Allison Janse, my wonderful, savvy, and patient editor, Kim Weiss, and everyone at HCI Books, thank you for being as passionate about this book as I am. Stephanie DeMizio, words cannot express my gratitude. You got this book off the ground. Thank you for your brilliant writing and editing. You gave my thoughts order and my book a voice. I could not have done this without you.

A huge thank you to Michele LoBosco for shooting the beauty looks. Your gorgeous images made my book so much prettier. I love working with you—you keep me on track and think of all the details.

A big shout-out to all the gorgeous models: Jennifer, Michelle, Anita, Liberty, Belen, Camille, Erika, Raye, Jaydn, Ani, and Nicole. You are all such pros. A huge thank you to Jona Tayor, my adorable niece, who documented the beauty shoot and stayed up all night with me organizing beauty looks. Deep gratitude goes to my fantastic assistant, Meghan Sanchez. Thank you for wearing a million hats and jumping in whenever and wherever I needed you to. You are the best. Brontë, Siyvan, and Sarah, your social media skills crushed it. Thank you for all your help with the book launch.

Don Flood, thank you for taking an amazing photo of me and allowing me to use it on the book cover. I am thrilled to be photographed by you. Much gratitude to Yeva Babayan who beautifully illustrated my book.

I am ever grateful to my agents, Madeline Leonard, Susanna Burke, and the CloutierRemix gang. Working with you has been an honor and a privilege. Ken Cook, thank your for giving the talk "Ten Americans" nearly a decade ago and educating me about chemicals in cosmetics. Nneka Leiba, your help and support with the database has made my job so much easier. Thank you. I am forever grateful to all the cosmetic companies who have supported me all these years.

A big hug to all my amazing friends: Dr. Richard McNabb, thank you for your critical eye, expert editing skills, and generously taking the time to read and edit the first draft of my proposal. I am so proud to call you my friend. Stacie Searcy-Ernsdorf, my deepest gratitude for your thorough reads and keen attention to detail on my proposal. Marianna and I count the days to your charitable Sunday morning visits. You are adored. Laura Connelly, a big kiss to you for your daily "check ins" on baby and me. Your girlfriend pep talks—you kept me sane. I cherish you. Thank you to your mom, Catherine, and Aunt Diana for including Marianna and me in all your lovely family gatherings. Lisa Carter, we have been through so much together—we have wonderful memories. Thank you for getting me out of the house for decadent dinners and catch-up sessions when I needed it most. Your friendship means the world to me. Ally Vickers, the best travel mate ever—we had such a blast. Thank you for your expert hair styling on the beauty looks and making me laugh. Nina Davis, my wise friend and sounding board, thank you for the marathon heart-to-hearts and words of wisdom throughout the years. You are an amazing friend. Erin Barrow, your free spirit inspires me. Thank you for dreaming big with me every day. Thank you to my dear friend Gina Nazzaro, my biggest cheerleader. I now understand what "checking in" means for I miss you every day. A huge thank you to Ruben Shakhnazaryan, whose late-night runs for baby Motrin and almond milk relieved me tremendously. I'm deeply grateful to you for always being there for me when I need you. You are a rock star. Thank you all for being part of our life.

Thank you to my family for a lifetime of support and encouragement. I am fortunate to have a large loving family (with too many to name individually) cheering me on. A special thanks to my Aunt Judy for always believing in me and instilling in me an amazing work ethic. Thank you from the bottom of my heart to my daughter's care-givers, Anaheit and Helen, and their families for taking such wonderful care of Marianna and making us part of your family. Without your care, flexibility, and support there would be no book.

Last, but certainly not least, thank you to Jillian Michaels for a decade of support not only as a client but as a friend. You are the absolute best "client" any makeup artist could ever wish for. You inspire me and gave me the courage to say "Why not me?" I appreciate you immensely. You are forever my hero.

Resources

Books

Beauty to Die For, Judi Vance

Cosmetics Unmasked, Dr. Stephen & Gina Antczak

Drop Dead Gorgeous, Kim Erickson

Gorgeous for Good, Sophie Uliano

Healthy Beauty, Samuel S. Epstein, MD

No More Dirty Looks, Siobhan O'Connor & Alexandra Spunt

Not Just a Pretty Face, Stacy Malkan

The Green Beauty Guide, Julie Gabriel

The Body Toxic, Nena Baker
The Honest Life, Jessica Alba

Green Beauty Websites

A Green Beauty Magazine *(http://www.agreenbeauty.com)*

Christy Coleman *(http://christycoleman.com)*

Indigo + Canary *(http://indigoandcanary.com)*

Kimberlyloc *(www.kimberlyloc.com)*

Live Pretty Naturally *(http://livingprettynaturally.com)*

Makeup by Mary B *(http://www.makeupbymaryb.com)*

Organic Beauty Blogger *(http://www.organicbeautyblogger.com)*

Organic Beauty Talk *(www.organicbeautytalk.com)*

Paige Padgett *(http://paigepadgett.com)*

The Clean Beauty Blog *(http://thecleanbeautyblog.tumblr.com)*

The Glamorganic Goddess *(http://www.glamorganicgoddess.com)*

The Green Beauty Team *(http://greenbeautyteam.com)*

The Natural Junkie *(http://www.thenaturaljunkie.com)*

Brands

100% Pure

AEOS

Acure

Alima Pure

Antonym Cosmetics

ama la

Arcona

Aubrey Organics

Beautycounter

Buddha Nose

Couleur Caramel

Crazy Rumors

Deborah Lippmann

Derma *e*

Dr. Alkaitis

Dr. Bronner's Soaps

Dr. Hauschka

Ecco Bella

Eco Lips

EcoTools

EO

Evan Healy

Farmaesthetics

Gabriel Cosmetics

GlamNatural

Hamandi

Honeybee Gardens

Honoré des Prés

Hynt Beauty

Ilia Beauty

Indie Lee

Inika

Intelligent Nutrients

Jane Iredale

John Masters Organics

Juice Beauty

Jurlique

Keri Gran

Kaer Weis

Kur by Londontown

Lavera Naturkosmetik

Logona Naturkosmetik

Luminance Skincare

May Lindstrom Skin

Miessence

Mineral Fusion

MyChelle Dermaceuticals

Naturopathica

Pacifica Beauty

Pangea Organics

PATYKA

Persephenie

Physicians Formula Organic Wear

Primitive

Priti NYC

Prtty Peaushun

Rare El'ements

Red Flower

Restorsea

Revolution Organics

RODIN Olio Lusso

S.W. Basics

Scotch Naturals

Sheswai Lacquer

SkinOwl

Soapwalla

Sodashi

SpaRitual

RMS Beauty

Suki

Soleo Organics

Tammy Fender

Tata Harper

Terra Firma Cosmetics

Tweezerman

Vapour Organic Beauty

Vive Sana

Weleda Hair

W3ll People Makeup

Yarok

Zoya

Zuii Organic

Zuzu Luxe

This is a partial brand list. Please see my website for a complete list and updates *www.PaigePadgett.com*

Notes

1   "Dermal Absorption," first draft prepared by Drs. Janet Kielhorn, Stephanie Melching-Kollmuß, and Inge Mangelsdorf, Environmental Health Criteria 235, World Health Organization; available at *http://www.who.int/ipcs/pub lications/ehc/ehc235.pdf?ua=1.*

2   "Why This Matters: Cosmetics and Your Health," EWG's Skin Deep Cosmetics Database, 2011; article available at *http://www.ewg.org/skindeep/2011 /04/12/why-this-matters/.*

3   See "Product Testing" under "Cosmetics" at the FDA website, along with related subjects: *http://www.fda.gov/cosmetics/scienceresearch/producttesting/.*

4   *Cancer.org,* Known and Probable Carcinogens, *http://www.cancer.org/ cancer/cancercauses/othercarcinogens/generalinformationaboutcarcinogens/ known-and-probable-human-carcinogens.*

5   See the IARC Monographs on the Evaluation of Carcinogenic Risks to Humans, IARC website, *http://monographs.iarc.fr/ENG/Classification/.*

6   See the complete list at *http://monographs.iarc.fr/ENG/Classification/Classifi cationsAlphaOrder.pdf.*

7   "Carcinogenic 1,4-Dioxane Found in Leading 'Organic' Brand Personal Care Products," Organic Consumers Association, *https://www.organicconsumers .org/old_articles/bodycare/DioxaneRelease08.php.*

8   "Study: Almost Half of All 'Natural' Personal Care Products Contain Known Carcinogen," Environmental Working Group, June 23, 2008, *http:// www.ewg.org/news/testimony-official-correspondence/study-almost-half-all- %E2%80%98natural%E2%80%99-personal-care-products.*

9   "Retinol (Vitamin A) for Anti-Aging," Paula's Choice, *http://www.paulas choice.com/expert-advice/anti-aging/_/retinol-for-anti-aging.*

10 State of California Environmental Protection Agency Office of Environmental Health Hazard Assessment Safe Drinking Water and Toxic Enforcement Act of 1986; Chemicals Known to the State to Cause Cancer or Reproductive Toxicity, March 27, 2015, *http://oehha.ca.gov/prop65/prop65_list/files/P65single 03272015.pdf.*

11 Eileen D. Kuempel and Avima Ruder, "Titanium Dioxide (TiO₂)," IARC Monograph 93, *http://monographs.iarc.fr/ENG/Publications/techrep42/TR42-4.pdf.*

12 "Sunbeds and UV Radiation," IARC, June 2009.

13 Vivian Diller, "8 Ways to Feel Beautiful from the Inside Out," *Oprah Winfrey Show*, September 2010, *http://www.oprah.com/oprahshow/8-Tips-on-Feeling-Beautiful-from-the-Inside-Out#ixzz3aLPiySiM.*

14 Benjamin S. Halpern et al., "A Global Map of Human Impact on Marine Ecosystems," *Science* 319, no. 5865 (February 2008): 948–52.

15 "The Reporting List of Chemicals of High Concern to Children (CHCC)," Children's Safe Products Act, Department of Ecology, State of Washington, *http://www.ecy.wa.gov/programs/swfa/cspa/chcc.html.*

16 Minnesota House Bill 458 (May 13, 2013); the ban was approved by a 113–13 vote.

About the Photographers and Illustrator

DON FLOOD is an accomplished celebrity photographer whose work has appeared in the pages of *Vanity Fair, Esquire, Italian Flair, French Glamour, In Style, Shape, Marie Claire* and many other publications. Flood has shot for clients such as Nexxus, Cover Girl, Clairol, Victoria's Secret and L'Oreal, and has shot everyone from Beyonce to Jennifer Lawrence and Britney Spears to Mary J. Blige, Ben Affleck, Naomi Watts and many others. In addition to his unparalleled photography, and when he's not designing for his wallcovering line, FLIEPAPER, Don is also a tennis player and an avid runner and has completed several marathons. Don lives near the beach in Santa Monica and has a weekend house in Palm Springs.

MICHELE LoBOSCO is a portrait and fashion photographer. She was born and raised in Brooklyn, but currently lives in Los Angles where she enjoys taking pictures of colorful characters and photographing fashion editorials. She's been published in numerous books and publications including *Fashion Gone Rogue, Creem, Cake, Bisous,* and *Status Magazine.* She lives in Venice Beach with her husband and much-loved pup, eating more pasta than she should and bike riding around on her pastel blue bicycle.

YEVA BABAYAN is an illustrator and a graphic artist currently living and working in Los Angeles. Her work is very much influenced from inspiration she draws from nature and her travels around the world. She is currently a senior designer with Kelly Wearstler, happily creating beautiful objects for the world to enjoy. You can see some of her creations at *www.yevalution.com.*

About the Author

PAIGE PADGETT, author and green beauty expert, has never been afraid to go against the grain. An irreverent, free spirit, she follows her instincts and her heart. At the mere age of twelve she announced to her family that she was no longer eating red meat. Ironically, her half–Native American grandfather was a cattle rancher. It was no surprise, then, that when beauty experts said she couldn't provide safe and eco-friendly makeup artistry and still create beautiful faces, she set out to prove them wrong—and did.

Now considered a leading authority on green beauty, Paige has been the Green Beauty Expert for Dasani ECOmmunity Facebook Page, DailyGlow.com, and the Jillian Michaels Wellness Team and founded Paigepadgett.com, a green beauty website. In addition, she is often sought out by the press and has been featured in *Shape, Elle, GenLux, Ladies Home Journal, The Los Angeles Times, Vegetarian Times, Natural Health* and *Whole Life Times Magazine*. Her television, radio, podcasts, and live appearances include "Martha Stewart Radio," "San Diego Live," "The Jillian Michaels Radio Show," "Green Is Good," "The Healthy Voyager," and "The Jillian Michaels Wellness Cruise."

Index